# Genetic Counseling and Preventive Medicine
## in Post-War Bosnia

Philip C. Aka

# Genetic Counseling and Preventive Medicine in Post-War Bosnia

palgrave
macmillan

Philip C. Aka
International University of Sarajevo
Sarajevo, Bosnia and Herzegovina

ISBN 978-981-15-7986-8          ISBN 978-981-15-7987-5   (eBook)
https://doi.org/10.1007/978-981-15-7987-5

This Palgrave Macmillan imprint is published by the registered company Springer Nature Singapore Pte Ltd.
The registered company address is: 152 Beach Road, #21-01/04 Gateway East, Singapore 189721, Singapore

*To my family, the memories of my father and of the inimitable Evangeline C. Aka. To the victims of the COVID-19 pandemic in Bosnia and Herzegovina and the rest of the world, for the teachable lessons in preventive medicine their infections and deaths hold for embattled healthcare systems across the globe. And to all my former students across the United States and southeastern Europe, for the opportunities that, semester after semester, they afforded me to learn with them.*

# PREFACE

This book contributes to the long-standing debate on healthcare reforms in Bosnia.[1] The debate reached a high point in September 2015 with the release of the document Reform Agenda for Bosnia and Herzegovina 2015–2018 by fourteen governments in Bosnia and Herzegovina. Thirteen of these governments comprise the Bosnian healthcare system. This contribution builds squarely around the concept of preventive medicine—quality medical attention short of complex examination and treatment, that is actuated by the need to remove the causes of ill-health. The book portrays preventive medicine as a function of progress in genetic counseling, plus alcohol and tobacco controls. More elaborately, the book's argument is that twenty-five years after the ethnic war that shook Bosnia and Herzegovina to its foundations at the dawn of its independent nationhood, healthcare reforms in the land is a function of preventive medicine, defined as genetic counseling, backed by tobacco and alcohol controls.

Self-reflectively, the book is a boon to comparative analysis and a tribute to the possibilities of research in the Information Age. First on comparative analysis, the book is a study of healthcare reforms in Bosnia set in the multidisciplinary field of Bioethics, supplemented by comparative healthcare studies, and comparative human right studies. The book taps into each of these multiple literatures while, simultaneously, contributing ideas from Bosnia into each literature. As a field of study, Bioethics is concerned with the ethical issues emerging from advances in biology and medicine, including the ethical questions that arise in the relationships among life sciences, biotechnology, medicine, politics, law, and philosophy. Bioethics "draw[s] attention to the fact that the rapid advances in science ha[ve] proceeded without due attention being paid to values."[2] Next on research possibilities in the Information Age, the book is based on an extensive list of electronically accessible literature on healthcare in English in the public domain. In addition to Bosnia, these materials encompass sources from the United States and Europe, including nations from former Yugoslavia now neighbors of Bosnia—all within the best tradition of comparative analysis and interdisciplinary studies.

It takes a village to raise a child.[3] Similarly, multiple sources inspired this book. Consistent with the metaphor of village, those sources may be called hamlets and villagers. Among the various hamlets, two here deserve special acknowledgment. The first is my presence in Bosnia and Herzegovina where, for nearly two and a half years, I maintained an academic home at the Law Faculty of the International University of Sarajevo (IUS) located in the Sarajevan suburb of Ilidža. This book spans and tracks my period there. The Igbo of West Africa have a saying that advises sojourners to strive to thrive in any location they happen to make their home. But for my residence in the Bosnian capital Sarajevo, I would not have had the motivation to write this book on healthcare reforms in Bosnia and Herzegovina. The second metaphorical hamlet needing acknowledgment in this book is the Southern Illinois University School of Law at Carbondale, Illinois (SIU Law), where I was a visiting professor in spring of 2020. The contract for this book was signed with Palgrave Macmillan in February, time enough before the global lockdown occasioned by the need to contain the spread of the COVID-19 pandemic, with its mayhem of infections and deaths.

At the IUS metaphorical hamlet, the villagers include Sabina Semiz and Sencer Yeralan. Sabina organized the roundtable on October 27, 2017, in commemoration of World Bioethics Day that year, where the earliest version of this topic was presented. Sabina also introduced me to the field of Bioethics, which progressed from an invitation into her course as a guest-lecturer in Fall of 2018, through my completing the class when she took ill toward the end of that semester, to our joint authorship in Fall of 2019 of a piece on precision medicine (genetic testing, counseling, and editing),[4] among the sources I have drawn upon in building my argument for preventive medicine in this book. Like Sabina, Yeralan helped deepen my interest in interdisciplinary studies all the way to the exploration and coauthorship of a piece on the possible benefits of humor as teaching tool in higher education in Bosnia.[5] Other villagers from the IUS hamlet include

Ahmet Yildirim, Rector, under whose leadership I served as dean of the Faculty of Law from 2018 to 2019, Ognjen Riđić, and Edin Ćatović. At SIU Law, the villagers worthy of appreciation are the entire faculty, under the leadership of Cindy Buys and Jennifer Brobst, for their cordiality.

Other villagers outside the narrow confines of IUS and SIU Law include Josh Pitt, senior commissioning editor at Palgrave Macmillan in charge of the Pivot program under which this book is published, and his assistant Charanya Manoharan. The contract for this book was signed and the manuscript concluded in the midst of the infections and deaths of COVID-19 while I was at Carbondale, Illinois. Thank you, Josh, for believing in this project and, along with Charanya, for goading me on to complete it timely when, amid saturated news of infections and deaths from the Coronavirus, I experienced occasional lapses in motivation for hard work. Gilbert Abraham, Osi(na)chi Aguocha, Obi Anaba, Okezie Anidobu, A.B. Assensoh, Joseph Balogun, Agber Dimah, Kenneth Ihenetu, Emmanuel Iheukwumere, Gary Kline, John Mukum Mbaku, Rev. Sister Francisca Nzeke, Sampson Onwueyi, Waren Tsafa, Hassan Wahab, and Musa Yahaya, you know your roles within the broader village and I appreciate each of you for your respective acts of support. Among others, I dedicate this book to a group of consummate villagers: the hundreds of students across the United States and Europe that I have taught in my over twenty-five years in higher education for the numerous opportunities that, semester after semester, they afforded me to learn with them. Consistent with academic canons, none of these villagers takes the blame for any errors in this work. A shorter version of this book appeared as an article in 50(2), 271–340, of the *California Western International Law Journal*, published in the spring of 2020. I also gratefully acknowledge the permission of Crisis Group to reproduce the map of Bosnia and Herzegovina on p. xvii.

Carbondale, IL, USA                                              Philip C. Aka
May 2020

## NOTES

1. On a note of style and for the sake of consistency, this book spells out "healthcare" as one word, except where quoting the work of other writers who break the term into two words. Likewise, the book spells "counseling"

with one "l," except where quoting the work of other writers who spell the term with two "ls."

2. UNESCO, Sector for Social and Human Sciences, *Bioethics Core Curriculum: Section 1: Syllabus Ethics Education Program* (2016), Unit 2, https://unesdoc.unesco.org/ark:/48223/pf0000246885

3. See Hilary Rodham Clinton, *It Takes a Village*, Tenth Anniversary Ed. (New York: Simon & Schuster, 2006 (1996)) (among other things, discussing the more or less positive impacts that individuals and groups in society outside the family have on a child's well-being). Following are two of the discussions specifically pertinent to this book: "An Ounce of Prevention is Worth a Pound of Intensive Care" (99–116), and "Let Us Build a Village Worthy of Our Children" (295–98). The inspiration for the analogy of a book to a child comes from the renowned Nigerian novelist Chinua Achebe (1930–2013). Asked about which of his novels he liked the most, Achebe responded that the question was a difficult one akin to asking a parent which of his children the parent loved the most. A thoughtful parent, he said, would respond in terms of the uniqueness of each child. Chinua Achebe, *Arrow of God* (Heinemann, 1964), book's preface.

4. Sabina Semiz & Philip C. Aka, "Precision Medicine in the Era of CRISPR-Cas9: Evidence from Bosnia and Herzegovina," 5 *Palgrave Communications* (2019), 134, https://doi.org/10.1057/s41599-019-0346-2

5. Philip C. Aka & Sencer Yeralan, "Humor as Pedagogy: Evidence from Bosnia and Herzegovina," *Indones. J. Int'l & Comp. Law*, VI (4), 539–603.

# CONTENTS

# ABBREVIATIONS

| | |
|---|---|
| BAM | Bosnian Convertible Mark, the Bosnian currency; see also KM |
| BiH | Bosnia and Herzegovina |
| COVID-19 | Name of the disease caused by the Coronavirus; declared by the World Health Organization as a pandemic |
| DALYs | Disability-adjusted life years |
| DNA | Deoxyribonucleic acid |
| DTC | Direct-to-consumer genetic test |
| DZ | Dom zdravlje (Croatian for "House of Health"). |
| FBiH | Federation of Bosnia and Herzegovina |
| GDP | Gross domestic product |
| HP | *Hitna pomoc*, Bosnian for ambulance |
| ICESCR | International Covenant on Economic, Social, and Cultural Rights |
| KM | Bosnian abbreviation for BAM |
| RS | Republika Srpska, one of the two entities that make up BiH |
| SDA | Party of Democratic Action (one of the leading political parties in Bosnia) |
| UNDP | United Nations Development Program, publisher of the Human Development Index, a UN publication published annually. |
| UNHCR | United Nations High Commissioner for Refugees |
| WHO | World Health Organization |
| ZAVNOBiH | *Zemaljsko antifašističko vijeće narodnog oslobođenja Bosne i Hercegovine* Bosnian for National Anti-Fascist Council of the People's Liberation of Bosnia and Herzegovina. |

# TABLE OF BOSNIAN NATIONAL AND
# INTERNATIONAL LAWS

Additional Protocol to the Convention on Human Rights and Biomedicine, Concerning Biomedical Research, C.E.T.S. No. 195 (January 9, 2007).

Constitution of Bosnia and Herzegovina. Annex 4 to the General Framework Agreement for Peace in Bosnia and Herzegovina. 1995.

Constitution of Republika Srpska. Official Gazette of the Republic of Srpska No. 21/92—Consolidated Version, 28/94, 8/96, 13/96, 15/96, 16/96, 21/96, 21/02, 26/02, 30/02, 31/02, 69/02, 31/03, 98/03, 115/05, 117/05, 48/11.

Convention for the Protection of Human Rights and Dignity of the Human Being with Regard to the Application of Biology and Medicine: Convention on Human Rights and Biomedicine (January 12, 1999), E.T.S. No. 16.

Council of Europe, Committee of Ministers, Recommendation No. R(92) 3 on Genetic Testing and Screening for Health Care Purposes (February 10, 1992)

Decision on the Base and Rate of Contribution for Health Insurance. Official Gazette of the Brčko District of BiH, 37/2009

European Social Charter (Revised), E.T.S. No. 163 (1996).

International Covenant on Economic, Social, and Cultural Rights. 1976. U.N. General Assembly Resolution No. 2200A (XXI) (December 19, 1966), 993 U.N.T.S. 3

The Law on Health Care. Official Gazette of the Federation of Bosnia and Herzegovina, No. 46/10, and 75/13

The Law on Health Care. Official Gazette of Republika Srpska, No. 18/99.

xvi TABLE OF BOSNIAN NATIONAL AND INTERNATIONAL LAWS

The Law on Health Insurance. Official Gazette of the Federation of Bosnia and Herzegovina, No. 30/97, 7/02, 70/08, and 48/11.

The Law on Health Insurance. Official Gazette of Republika Srpska, No. 18/99.

Ustav Socijalisticke Federativne Republike Jugoslvije [Constitution of the Socialist Federal Republic of Yugoslavia], 1974

Vienna Convention on the Law of Treaties, *opened for signature* May 23, 1969, 1115 U.N.T.S. 331.

Statute of the Brčko District of Bosnia and Herzegovina. Office of the High Representative, 1999.

# MAP OF BOSNIA AND HERZEGOVINA

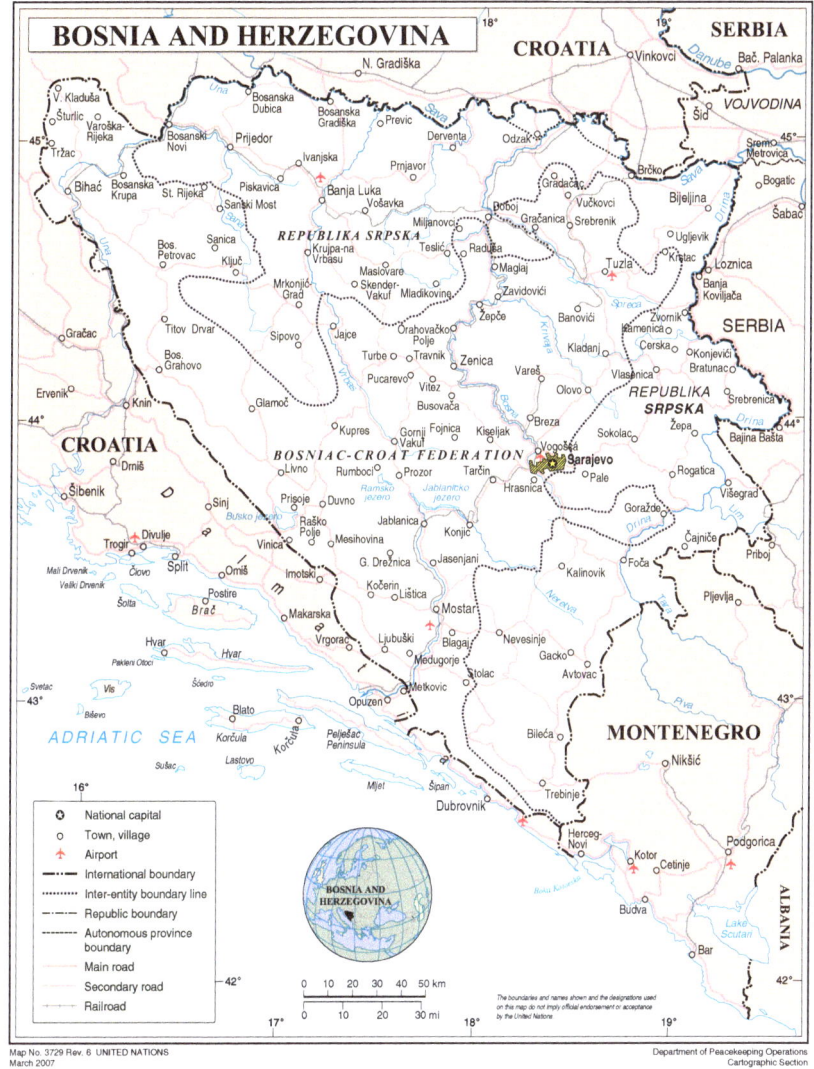

# LIST OF TABLES

# CHAPTER 1

# Introduction

**Abstract** This chapter provides a statement relating to the debate on healthcare reforms in Bosnia, including a primer on the country, the argument of the study, and the book's organization.

**Keywords** Healthcare in Bosnia's Reform Agenda • Genetic counseling • Preventive medicine • Bioethics • Comparative healthcare studies • Comparative human right studies

## PRIMER ON BOSNIA AND HERZEGOVINA

Bosnia and Herzegovina (BiH)[1] is a state of two entities, plus a self-governing unit, a federation of sorts, dominated by three ethnic communities.[2] Geographically speaking, BiH is located in south-eastern Europe, west of the Balkan Peninsula.[3] With a landmass of 51,197 square kilometers, BiH is comparable in size to the State of West Virginia in the United States (62,758 square kilometers), Croatia (56,594 square kilometers), and Slovakia (49,035 square kilometers).[4] The country is bordered by Croatia to the north, Serbia and Montenegro to the east, and the Adriatic Sea to the south, with a total boundary length of 1389 kilometers.[5]

BiH has a population of 3.5 million people.[6] The figure is 1 million people less than 4.5 million persons from the prewar census in 1991.[7] The significant drop in population is due to various factors, including a negative perception of their socioeconomic futures by many Bosnians and a

1
P. C. Aka, *Genetic Counseling and Preventive Medicine in Post-War Bosnia*, https://doi.org/10.1007/978-981-15-7987-5_1

fertility rate below replacement numbers.[8] Bosnia is a post-socialist state with a service-based economy.[9] It is one of six components of former Socialist Federal Republic of Yugoslavia (SFRY).[10] SFRY existed from 1945 to 1992, although its roots date back to the Kingdom of Serbs, Croats, and Slovens, formed in December of 1918.[11] Bosnians' self-awareness of their separate statehood goes back in time to the tenth century.[12] One recent expression of this self-image was in 1943 when BiH's present boundaries were determined as part of a boundary-making exercise for the whole of Yugoslavia.[13]

## HEALTHCARE IN BOSNIA'S REFORM AGENDA

In September of 2015, fourteen governments which make up Bosnia and Herzegovina drew up a set of proposals for reform in several fields of national development that included healthcare.[14] The fourteen governments were the Council of Ministers of Bosnia and Herzegovina, the Government of the Federation of Bosnia and Herzegovina (FBiH),[15] the Government of Republika Srpska (RS), the Government of Brčko District, and the governments of the ten Cantons in FBiH—Una-Sana, Posavina, Tuzla, Zenica-Doboj, Bosnia-Podrinje, Central Bosnia, Herzegovina-Neretva, West Herzegovina, Sarajevo, and Canton 10 (West Bosnia Canton).[16] The fourteen governmental units, minus the Council of Ministers of Bosnia and Herzegovina, constitute the BiH healthcare system, itself alternatively organized around two entities, plus a self-governing unit—FBiH and its ten Cantons, RS, and Brčko District.[17]

Broadly, the fourteen governments "recognize[d] an urgent need to initiate a process of rehabilitating and modernizing the economy with a view to" realizing certain cherished values, such as "fostering sustainable, efficient, socially[-]just and steady economic growth; [and] creating new jobs[.]"[18] With specific reference to healthcare, the fourteen governments pledged to curtail "the burden on labor needs" "by reducing contributions for health insurance, coupled at the same time with the need to ensure additional revenues for extra-budgetary funds to cover the losses generated as a result of the reduced contribution rate."[19] The team of fourteen governments also pledged to "seek financial and technical assistance [from] the World Bank to implement" several aspects of healthcare reform, "includ[ing] a solution for outstanding debts," and defining "new models and sources of funding, with a more precise regulation of the network of health care institutions."[20] Finally, the fourteen governments proposed to "support an increase in excise duties on tobacco and alcohol which will be the direct income of the health insurance fund of the RS and health insurance funds in the FBiH, Cantons[,] and Brčko District by the end of 2015."[21] These pledges of healthcare reform culminated "an increased demand from many sectors for improved and comprehensive information on the workings and quality of the health care system in Bosnia and Herzegovina," the Office of the United Nations High Commissioner for Refugees (UNHCR) in Sarajevo commented upon in a study that the office published in 2001.[22]

## Argument

This book contributes to the long-standing debate on healthcare reforms that reached a high point in the Reform Agenda for BiH discussed in the previous section. Bosnia is a nation forged in war.[23] Twenty-five years after the bloody fighting, Bosnians have yet to recover fully from the war that shook the country to its very foundation on the verge of its nationhood.[24] The contribution to the debate on healthcare reforms this book embodies revolves around the concept of preventive medicine—quality medical attention short of complex examination and treatment, that is actuated by the need to remove the causes of ill-health.[25] The book portrays preventive medicine as a function of progress in genetic counseling,[26] plus alcohol and tobacco controls.[27] More elaborately, the book's argument is that twenty-five years after the ethnic war that shook Bosnia and Herzegovina to its foundations at the dawn of its independent nationhood, healthcare reforms in the land is a function of preventive medicine, defined as genetic counseling, backed by alcohol and tobacco controls.[28]

BiH maintains an abiding commitment to socioeconomic human rights, including healthcare, that dates back to its socialist incarnation in Yugoslavia.[29] However, *enjoyment* of these rights by citizens, particularly the healthcare rights at the focus of this book, lacks depth.[30] This is due to multiple forces which individually and collectively took a decided toll on these guarantees. Predictions are hazardous and this book takes no cause-and-effect position on the matter, but a foundational factor was the destruction of health and other infrastructure by the internecine war from 1992 to 1995 that convulsed BiH.[31] About 200,000 people died during the war with another 240,000 wounded, many of them seriously, some to the point of permanent disability.[32] Many of these were healthcare workers.[33] The war also devastated much of the country's already-modest healthcare infrastructure.[34] Problems after the war with negative ramifications for healthcare, including genetic testing and counseling at the heart of this study, revolved around deficiencies in the various hallmarks of a good healthcare system,[35] that this book pulls together in Chap. 4.

In the light of the foregoing, it may be argued that the quantity and quality of healthcare services produced today in BiH fall below "the facilities available in Western Europe" and the level achieved before the war.[36] First, the level of healthcare services provided to insured persons falls below the level guaranteed by law.[37] Second, despite the promise of an unalienable right to healthcare, a large number of the populace lack access to healthcare services, either because they do not have insurance or because they have insurance but experience difficulty accessing healthcare.[38] Third, healthcare financing in the country is marked by unabated deficits, which threaten the integrity and sustainability of the healthcare systems.[39] These deficits, "outstanding debts" as the Reform Agenda for BiH called them,[40] are piling up at a time of increased public demands for healthcare services, driven by rising expectations for these services.[41] A range of forces fueled this increased demand for healthcare services: an increase in the number of chronic diseases;[42] increased information availability and awareness; "new needs for health services," attributable to "the continuing development of medical technology";[43] among others.[44]

A stitch in time saves nine, as one adage goes;[45] preventive medicine is an idea whose time has come in Bosnia. One way that BiH leaders can help optimize *enjoyment* of healthcare benefits in this country is through relatively inexpensive means intrinsic to healthcare like genetic counseling. The emphasis nowadays in many healthcare systems, developed and developing alike, is primary healthcare, analogized to medical attention short of complex examination and treatment that does not sacrifice quality.[46] It is what the World Health Organization (WHO)[47] defines as "the first level of contact of individuals, the family and community with the national health system [...] and [...] the first element of a continuing health care process."[48] Preventive medicine pursued through means like genetic counseling arguably falls into that first element of a continuing healthcare process. It equally meets the requirement of the European Social Charter mandating state parties "to remove as far as possible the causes of ill health."[49] Moreover, the fear sometimes expressed that individuals at risk of inheriting a genetic disorder may feel a lack of perceived control over an affected risk if they performed a susceptibility testing has been found to be overblown.[50]

Recent epidemiological developments lend added credence and urgency to the theme of preventive medicine at the heart of this book. One such outbreak currently raging through all four geographic corners of the globe is the COVID-19 pandemic, theorized to be caused by the new Coronavirus.[51] The inadequate responses of many countries to the pandemic, more so by developing nations like Bosnia and Herzegovina,[52] underscore the need for stronger healthcare systems in these countries that are more responsive to health emergencies in an increasingly interconnected and interdependent international community.[53]

Self-reflectively, this book is a boon to comparative analysis.[54] The book is a study of healthcare reforms in Bosnia set in the multidisciplinary field of Bioethics, supplemented by comparative healthcare studies, and comparative human right studies. From these various fields, this case study on healthcare reforms in Bosnia taps themes in the process of developing independent ideas from the country that it then contributes to these fields.

## GENETIC COUNSELING EMBEDDED IN PREVENTIVE MEDICINE AS DEFINED IN THIS STUDY

Genetic counseling is defined in Chap. 5 of this book. Anticipating that conversation, rather than preempting it, it is important to stress at this point that a fine line arguably separates genetic counseling from the broader species enhancement techniques like eugenics[55] or gene editing.[56] In the non-expansive sense it is used in this book, *genetic counseling* is the process by which patients and families at risk of an inherited disorder receive tailored advice (counseling) related to that disorder to minimize the chances of transmitting such disorder to future generations.[57] It is preventive medicine designed to catch a problem at an early stage before it festers and assumes hydra-headed dimension(s) that may necessitate the channel or allocation of scarce healthcare resources in an (after-the-fact) attempt to resolve it. It does *not* include broader species enhancement techniques, inconsistent with the tenets of Bioethics, a field of study which works to check some of the worst excesses of modern scientific discoveries.[58]

As the Council of Europe advised, genetic testing must be a "non-directive" procedure, "adapted to the circumstances in which individuals and families receive genetic information," and "accompanied by appropriate counselling, both before and after the procedure."[59] The academic literature identifies three aspects to genetics embedded in precision or personalized medicine: genetic testing, genetic counseling, and gene editing.[60] As used here, *genetic counseling* encompasses the first two categories and excludes the third, specifically the inappropriate use of innovative editing techniques to alter human deoxyribonucleic acid (DNA).[61]

Finally, the focus in this book is limited to genetic tests conducted in an approved clinical setting.[62] These tests meet the prescriptions of the Council of Europe relating to approval by a competent state authority and participation in an "external quality assurance."[63] The focus does not include tests which lack these clinical features—such as those undertaken by testing companies which, because they ply their products directly to their customers, are known colloquially as direct-to-consumer (DTC) genetic testing companies. DTC companies "stress[] the 'informational' and 'fun' aspects of their services" of such manner that some critics believe "underplay[] the health implications of their services."[64] These tests raise issues of effective regulation domestically and internationally outside the scope of this book.[65] More discussion on the concept and clinical practice of genetic counseling is saved for Chap. 5 devoted to that topic.

## ORGANIZATION OF THIS BOOK

Using the technique of preventive medicine embedded in the "ounce" of genetic counseling, this book contributes answers to the "demand for improved and comprehensive information on the workings and quality of the health care system in" BiH.[66] From a policy standpoint, stitch-in-time, the vernacular of preventive medicine, that drives this book, is more than a proverb; it is instructively a call-out to Bosnian policymakers, in partnership with other stakeholders, including international agencies, to implement a timely and relatively economically painless stitch in preventive medicine that saves nine for a resource-poor, post-conflict society. The prescriptive tone syncs with the inherent normative tone of comparative healthcare studies.[67]

The book comprises eight chapters, in three parts, including this introduction as Chap. 1. Part I dealing with threshold issues comprises Chaps. 2 and 3. Chapter 2 provides the background history related to the topic embedded in an abstract commitment to healthcare as socioeconomic human rights, cemented in constitutional documents all the way from socialist Yugoslavia. Chapter 3 describes the features of the Bosnian healthcare system, comprising the two complementary issues of its characteristic features and levels of healthcare delivery service. Part II on healthcare reforms as human right comprises one chapter, Chap. 4, which lays out four hallmarks of a good healthcare system as guide to healthcare reforms in Bosnia. The hallmarks are human right-sensitive benchmarks that mimic some of the measurement tools in the academic literature on comparative healthcare studies,[68] including concepts and materials from a seminal study by the World Health Organization in 2000.[69] Part III titled "Toward Preventive Medicine in BiH" comprises three complementary chapters: Chap. 5 consisting of a statement on the definition of genetic counseling; Chap. 6 presenting the status of genetic counseling in the Bosnian healthcare system; and Chap. 7 highlighting measures that could be used to achieve preventive medicine in BiH through genetic counseling, backed by tobacco and alcohol controls. Chapter 8 concludes the work in a discussion that reflects on the significance of this study not only for the interdisciplinary field of Bioethics wherein this book is set, but also for the two complementary fields of comparative healthcare studies, and comparative human right studies.

## NOTES

1. The abbreviation is Bosnian for Bosnia i Hercegovina. The author prefers it over two competing acronyms: "B&H," given the awkwardness of the ampersand in the coinage; and over "BH" which elides the "and." BiH is occasionally alternated in this book with Bosnian. This is a term of adjectival and/or adverbial convenience that, rather than designate only Bosnians (one of the major ethnic groups in BiH), instead encompasses all citizens, including Croats and Serbs, the two other major ethnic groups of the country. In other words, although technically inaccurate, in the sense it is used in this book, the designation is informal, and there is no suggestion that it is the exact equivalent or substitute for the full name.

2. Federation of sorts because power is decentralized in one of the two entities that make up the country, the Federation of Bosnia and Herzegovina (FBiH), while relatively centralized in the other, Republika Srpska (RS). FBiH makes up 51% of the country's landmass and is controlled by Bosniaks and Croats, while RS constitutes 49% of the territory and is controlled by Serbs. The self-governing unit, belonging to both entities, rather than controlled by any of them, is Brčko District, established on March 8, 2000, in the aftermath of the civil war in the country from April 1992 to December 1995. Classified based on religious affiliation, Bosniaks are overwhelmingly Muslims, Croats Catholics, and Serbs Orthodox

Christians. For more or less elaborate overview of the BiH political system, see Saša Gavrić et al., *The Political System of Bosnia and Herzegovina: Institutions, Actors, Processes* (Sarajevo Open Center, 2013); and Michaela Führer, *Bosnia-Herzegovina's Political System*, DW (Oct. 25, 2011), https://www.dw.com/en/bosnia-herzegovinas-political-system/a-15486583, *archived at* https://perma.cc/GT9X-ZMT. For an insightful discussion on the evolution of BiH federalism, including the studied choice of the framers of the 1995 Constitution to minimize portrayal of the country as a federal system, see Soeren Keil, "Federalism as a Tool of Conflict-Resolution: The Case of Bosnia and Herzegovina," 1(363) *Dans L'Europe en Formation* [*Europe in Formation*] 1(363) (2012): 205, https://www.cairn.info/revue-l-europe-en-formation-2012-1-page-205.htm

3. Depending on who is doing the counting and analysis, the Balkan Peninsula and region comprises ten or eleven political communities: Albania, Bulgaria, Croatia, Greece, Kosovo, Montenegro, North Macedonia, Romania, Serbia, Slovenia, and, for some analysts, Turkey. Along with BiH, some of these territories—Croatia, Kosovo, North Macedonia, Serbia, and Slovenia—were part of the former Yugoslavia. See Richard J. Crampton, "Balkans," *Encyclopedia Britannica*, https://www.britannica.com/place/Balkans

4. "Bosnia and Herzegovina: Location, Size, and Extent," *Nations Encyclopedia*, http://www.nationsencyclopedia.com/Europe/Bosnia-and-Herzegovina-LOCATION-SIZE-AND-EXTENT.html, *archived at* https://perma.cc/V5CH-FWXW

5. Ibid.

6. "Bosnia and Herzegovina," *Worldometer* (April 27, 2019), http://www.worldometers.info/world-population/bosnia-and-herzegovina-population/, *archived at* https://perma.cc/CJH7-3C7. Based on the latest 2013 census, the most numerous of the three largest ethnic groups are Bosniaks, who comprised 50.11% of the population, compared to Serbs 30.78%, and Croats 15.43%. See Rodolfo Toè, "Census Reveals Bosnia's Changed Demography," *BalkanInsight* (June 30, 2016), https://balkaninsight.com/2016/06/30/new-demographic-picture-of-bosnia-finally-revealed-06-30-2016/, *archived at* https://perma.cc/35DB-T2YZ

7. See Jennifer Cain et al., eds., *Health Care Systems in Transition: Bosnia and Herzegovina* (Copenhagen: European Observatory on Health Care Systems, 2002), 3. *See also* "Bosnia-Herzegovina Has Lost a Fifth of Its Pre-War Population, Census Shows," *Guardian* (London) (July 1, 2016), https://www.theguardian.com/world/2016/jul/01/bosnia-herzegovina-has-lost-a-fifth-of-its-pre-war-population-census-shows (story initially carried by *Agence France-Presse*). As of this headcount, 43.7% of the population identified themselves as Bosniaks, 31.3% as Serbs, and 17.3% as Croats. Cain et al., eds., note 7.

8. *See* Tim Judah, "Bosnia Powerless to Halt Demographic Decline," *BalkanInsight* (Nov. 21, 2019), https://balkaninsight.com/2019/11/21/bosnia-powerless-to-halt-demographic-decline/

9. Based on GDP share, in 2017 the economy of the country broke down into the following: little over 64% service activities, approximately 29% industry, and approximately 7% agriculture. See "Bosnia and Herzegovina," *CIA World Factbook* (updated Sept. 24, 2019), https://www.cia.gov/library/publications/the-world-factbook/geos/bk.html

10. The others, alphabetically, were Croatia, Macedonia, Montenegro, Serbia, and Slovenia, plus two autonomous provinces, Voljvodina and Kosovo, subsumed under Serbia. See, for example, Tomasz Bichta, ed., *Political Systems of the Former Yugoslavia: Bosnia and Herzegovina, Croatia, Kosovo, Macedonia, Montenegro, Servia, and Slovenia* (New York: Peter Lang, 2018).

11. See, for example, John R. Lampe & John B. Allcock, "Yugoslavia: Former Federated Nation (1929–2003)," *Encyclopedia Britannica*, https://www.britannica.com/place/Yugoslavia-former-federated-nation-1929-2003, archived at https://perma.cc/Q2FB-8TL4

12. Cain et al., eds., note 7, p. 3.

13. November 25 is observed as Statehood Day in BiH to commemorate the day in 1943 the ZAVNOBiH, legislative body of the Federal State of Bosnia and Herzegovina, then comprising 173 councilors, made a resolution which expressed the will of BiH as a distinct entity. ZAVNOBiH is a precursor of the BiH National Assembly. The declaration became law in 1995, vide The Law on the Proclamation of 25 November as the Statehood Day of Bosnia and Herzegovina, BiH Official Gazette No. 9/95, which sets aside November 25 as the Statehood Day of Bosnia and Herzegovina. However, the law is observed only in FBiH, not in RS. Statehood Day should *not* be confused with BiH's Independence Day, held each year on March 1 in honor of the controversial plebiscite in 1992 (63.6% of the population approved, less than the two-third majority necessary for the passage of a referendum) for the country's independence. See, for example, "Remembering Generation that Rebuilt Our Country: Happy Statehood Day of BiH!" *Sarajevo Times* (Nov. 29, 2019), https://www.sarajevotimes.com/remembering-generation-that-rebuilt-our-country-happy-statehood-day-of-bih-2/

14. See Reform Agenda for Bosnia and Herzegovina 2015–2018 (Working Translation) [hereinafter Reform Agenda for BiH], http://europa.ba/wp-content/uploads/2015/09/Reform-Agenda-BiH.pdf. (accessed July 22, 2019) (set of seventeen proposals, first seven of which are measures of fiscal consolidation and the last ten of which are classified into six structural areas of importance: public finance, taxation and fiscal sustainability; busi-

ness climate and competitiveness; labor market; social welfare and pension reform; rule of law and good governance; and public administration reform).

15. The abbreviation of this unit includes an "i" in place of "and" for the same reason indicated in note 1 with respect to the state-level government.
16. Reform Agenda for BiH, note 14, ¶ 1.
17. The fact that both technically and substantively the state-level government is no part of the BiH healthcare system is an odd impression that this book returns to later in Chaps. 4 and 7.
18. Reform Agenda for BiH, note 14, ¶ 1. The document disclosed that "[c]oncrete actions aimed at fiscal and financial sustainability and socio-economic reform will be augmented by targeted measures: to strengthen the rule of law and the fight against corruption; and to strengthen administrative capabilities and increase efficiency in public institutions at all [fourteen] levels of government." *Id.*
19. Reform Agenda for BiH, note 14, ¶ 8.
20. Ibid.
21. Ibid.
22. Werner Blatter, "Foreword and Acknowledgments," *in* United Nations High Commissioner for Refugees' Office of the Chief of Mission in Bosnia, *Health Care in Bosnia and Herzegovina in the Context of the Return of Refugees and Displaced Persons* (Sarajevo: Jul. 2001), https://www.unhcr. org/news/updates/2001/7/3c614f6a4/health-care-bosnia-herzegov-ina-context-return-refugees-displaced-persons.html [hereinafter *Health Care in BiH*]. At the time of this report, Blatter was chief of UNHCR Mission in BiH.
23. See Marcus Tanner, *Croatia: A Nation Forged in War* (New Haven, CT: Yale University Press, 3d Edition, 2010) (referring to Croatia, although, no different from its neighbor Croatia, Bosnia was also a nation forged in war).
24. Sarah A. Khan, "Bosnian Resurrection," *Arkansas Democrat Gazette* (July 7, 2019), https://www.arkansasonline.com/news/2019/jul/07/resur-rection-20190707/; Sarah Khan, "Bosnia and Herzegovina: Still Fighting But This Time for Life," *Independent* (UK), May 28, 2019, https://www. independent.co.uk/travel/bosnia-and-herzegovina-war-new-life-travel-visit-a8925981.html
25. See notes 45 and 48.
26. The term is defined in Chap. 5.
27. Tobacco and alcohol consumption are just two out of many environmental scourges that Bosnians endure. The Reform Agenda for BiH referenced these two. It talked about supporting an increase in excise duties on tobacco and alcohol which generates proceeds that go into the insurance

funds of FBiH and RS, as well as that of Brčko District. Reform Agenda for BiH, note 14, ¶ 8. Similarly, in their proposals for healthcare reforms, Marko Martić & Ognjen Đukić wrote about "new excise duties on tobacco, alcohol, fuel, harmful soft drinks, and luxur[y] products." Marko Martić & Ognjen Đukić, *Friedrich Ebert Stiftung Sarajevo,* "Health Care Systems in BiH: Financing Challenges and Reform Options?" (Oct. 2017), 28, https://library.fes.de/pdf-files/bueros/sarajevo/14124.pdf. In 2015, the number of deaths from ambient particulate air pollution, in absolute terms, was 2800. "Bosnia and Herzegovina: Absolute Number of Deaths from Ambient Particulate Air Pollution, 1990 to 2015," *Our World in Data,* https://ourworldindata.org/grapher/absolute-number-of-deaths-from-ambient-particulate-air-pollution?tab=chart&country=BIH. For the same year, the death rate from air pollution per 100,000 persons was over 82. "Bosnia and Herzegovina: Death Rate from Air Pollution (Per 100,000), 1990 to 2015," *Our World in Data,* https://ourworldindata. org/grapher/death-rate-from-air-pollution-per-100000?country=BIH (the precise number was 82.3%). Finally, around fall every year, four out of every five residents of the country follow the "weather" electronically or on TV. More often than not their main concern is the air pollution that hits the country around this time of the year. See Svetlana Javanović, "Sarajevo World's Most Polluted City, Poor Air Quality Seen Across Western Balkans," *Balkan Green Energy News* (Dec. 4, 2018), https://balkan-greenenergynews.com/sarajevo-worlds-most-polluted-city-poor-air-quality-seen-across-western-balkans/. For this insight, the author is indebted to Edin Ćatović, Administrative Manager, Technical Services, at the International University of Sarajevo.

28. Diagrammatically, the relationship may be depicted as follows: HCR in BiH = PM + TC + AC, where HCR stands for healthcare reforms, PM for preventive medicine, TC tobacco control, and AC alcohol control.

29. See Chap. 2 (6) (tracing the background history of healthcare in BiH).

30. See Chap. 3 (analyzing the features of the healthcare system in BiH).

31. See John R. Lampe, "Bosnian War: European History [1992–1995]," *Encyclopedia Britannica,* https://www.britannica.com/event/Bosnian-War. For studies on the Bosnian war, see, for example, Stephen L. Burg & Paul S. Shoup, *The War in Bosnia-Herzegovina: Ethnic Conflict and International Intervention* (Armonk NY: M.E. Sharpe, 2d ed. 1999); and Carole Rogel, *The Breakup of Yugoslavia and the War in Bosnia* (Westport, CT: Greenwood Publishing Group, 1998).

32. See Cain et al., eds., note 7, p. 10 (calculating the number of the dead at 140,000–200,000 people and the wounded at between 70,000 and 240,000).

33. Ibid., p. 17 (disclosing that "[a]round 30% of practicing health professionals were lost," through either casualties or migration).

34. Ibid. (disclosing that "about 30% of health facilities were destroyed or heavily damaged during the war," and that only 46 of the 80 emergency clinics in the country before 1992 survived the war). See also Stephen J. Kunitz, "The Making and Breaking of Yugoslavia and Its Impact on Health," *Am. J. Public Health*, 94(11) (November 2004), 1894 (arguing that the impact of the disintegration of Yugoslavia on the public health systems, including healthcare, "has been profound," in that, among other things, "[i]mproving and converging measures of mortality before the collapse gave way to increasing disparities afterward."); and M. Carballo et al., "Development of an Essential Drug List for Bosnia and Herzegovina," *J. Royal Society of Medicine*, 90 (Jun. 1997), 331–33, http://europepmc. org/backend/ptpmcrender.fcgi?accid=PMC1296311&blobtype=pdf. (discussing the negative impacts of the war on the healthcare system, including healthcare infrastructure).

35. The notation "good healthcare system" is a prescriptive usage in sync with the inherent normative tone of comparative healthcare studies. See Marc J. Roberts et al., *Getting Health Reform Right: A Guide to Improving Performance and Equity* (New York: Oxford University Press, 2008), 40–60 (commenting on the inescapable ethics of *appraising* national performance in healthcare). The same ethics is indicated by the value reference in several parts of this book, especially in Chap. 4, which spells out the hallmarks of a good healthcare system as a guide to healthcare reforms.

36. *Health Care in BiH,* note 22, p. i (Executive Summary), p. 25.

37. Ibid., p. 23.

38. Ibid. See also Chap. 4 (especially the section on inadequate healthcare funding in Bosnia).

39. Martić & Đukić, note 27, p. 20.

40. See note 20 and accompanying text.

41. Martić & Đukić, note 27, pp. 11, 13.

42. Ibid., p. 24.

43. Ibid., p. 13.

44. This residual factor is the moral hazard argument. It is what Martić and Đukić called "the habit of irrational use of health care services [among the populace], without taking into account the financial capabilities of the previous and the current systems of public health care in BiH," alternately elaborating that "unlimited access to all services provided in the area of primary health care, a large number of specialist consultancy diagnostic services, hospital treatment in the country and abroad, spa facilities, hospitalization and a number of other health services, were available to the population at the time of [former Yugoslavia]." Ibid. "Under the doctrine of

moral hazard in behavioral economics, a person or group of persons take risks without having to suffer [the] consequences" of their risky behavior. See Will Kenton & Brian Abbott, "Moral Hazard," *Investopedia*, https://www.investopedia.com/terms/m/moralhazard.asp, *archived at* https://perma.cc/Z9XK-NAKJ. For a refutation of this doctrine in the context of BiH, see Muhamed Saric & Victor G. Rodwin, "The Once and Future Health System in the Former Yugoslavia: Myths and Realities," *Journal of Public Health*, 14(2) (1993), 220, https://www.nyu.edu/projects/rodwin/future.html (contesting three images that the authors argue "[m]ost of the existing literature on the organization and financing of Yugoslavia's health system perpetuated").

45. James Baquet, "A Stitch in Time Saves Nine," *Shenzhen Daily* (Nov. 11, 2010), http://www.szdaily.com/content/2010-11/11/content_507 3819.htm, archived at https://perma.cc/Z9WZ-C5J6. Or, as the American founding father Benjamin Franklin (1706–1790) equally memorably put it, "[a]n ounce of prevention is better than a pound of cure." Quoted in Tara Craig, "Healthcare Marketing Compliance in the UK—Prevention Beats Cure," *PMLive* (July 1, 2014), https://www.pmlive.com/pharma_intelligence/healthcare_marketing_compliance_in_the_uk_-prevention_beats_cure_581532, archived at https://perma.cc/BPW7-EZ33

46. See *Health Care in BiH,* note 22, p. 12. The concept of preventive medicine here calls to mind the kid animal song lyric about five little monkeys who jumped on the bed. Each of the five bumped its head, and on each occasion Mama monkey dutifully called the doctor, who in each instance administered a preventive medicine: no more monkeys jumping on the bed. Intriguingly, each of the five ignored the advice, whereupon, with the fifth also—predictably—bumping its head, the doctor advised that all five monkeys be put to bed. Preventive medicine seems so basic, yet for some reason is also easily oversighted.

47. The WHO is a, if not the, global healthcare czar. Founded on April 7, 1948, the day set aside as World Health Day, the WHO directs and coordinates international health within the United Nations system. World Health Organization, *About WHO*, http://www.who.int/about/en/. See also Kelley Lee, *Global Institutions: The World Health Organization (WHO)* (Abingdon: Routledge, 2008); Gian Luca Burci & Claude-Henri Vignes, *World Health Organization* (Zuidpoolsingel, Netherlands: Kluwer Law Int'l, 2004). BiH became a member of this body following its admission into the United Nations on May 22, 1992. Bosnia and Herzegovina & UN, BHMissionUN, https://bhmissionun.org/bosnia-and-herzegovina-un-3/, archived at https://perma.cc/4TD4-4PX3.

48. World Health Organization, Declaration of Alma Ata, Int'l Conference on PHC [Primary Health Care], Alma-Ata, USSR (6–12 Sept. 1978), art. VI, http://www.who.int/publications/almaata_declaration_en.pdf. Arguably, primary healthcare goes deeper than this. The Int'l Conference on Primary Health Care in Alma-Atta identified eight essential elements of primary healthcare that in their thoroughgoingness range beyond basic healthcare. These elements were as follows: education concerning prevailing health problems and methods for addressing them; promoting food supply and proper nutrition; providing an adequate supply of safe water and basic sanitation; and maternal and child healthcare, including family planning. World Health Organization, *World Health Report 1995: Bridging the Gaps* (Geneva, 1995), 88 (box), https://www.who.int/whr/1995/en/whr95_en.pdf?ua=1 [hereinafter *World Health Report 1995*]. Others are immunization against the major infectious diseases, prevention and control of locally endemic diseases, appropriate treatment of common diseases and injuries, and providing essential drugs. Ibid.

49. European Social Charter (Revised), ETS No. 163 (1996), art. 11(1), rm. coe.int/168007cf93. BiH ratified the instrument in 2008, but accepts only 51 out of the 98 paragraphs of the agreement. Council of Europe, Bosnia and Herzegovina and the European Social Charter [Factsheet] (updated Mar. 2019), rm.coe.int/pdf/1680492808, archived at https://perma.cc/YV7U-VEVL. The provisions BiH does not accept include the system of collective complaints contained in an Additional Protocol of 1995 that it did not ratify. This means that only eligible nongovernmental organizations, not individuals, might lodge complaints regarding governmental compliance with the Charter.

50. See R.E. Collins et al., "Impact of Communicating Personalized Genetic Risk Information on Perceived Control Over the Risk: A Systematic Review," *Genetics in Medicine: Official J. American College of Medical Genetics*, 13(4) (2011), 273–7 (showing that there is little evidence supporting the fear that feedback of personalized genetic risk information may lead to "fatalism," defined as a lack of perceived control over the risk). See also Lejla Mahmutovic et al., "Perceptions of Students in Health and Molecular Life Sciences Regarding Pharmacogenomics and Personalized Medicine," *Human Genomics*, 12(1) (2018), 50 (reporting the results from a survey of 559 students from biomedical fields which indicated "a positive attitude of biomedical students in Bosnia and Herzegovina toward genetic testing[.]").

51. See "Q & A on Coronaviruses (COVID-19)," *World Health Org.*, who.int/news-room/q-a-detail/q-a-coronaviruses, *archived at* https://perma.cc/3UNS-L92T

52. See Nidzara Ahmetasevic, "Bosnia and Herzegovina's COVID-19 Response Threatens Fragile Human Rights," K2.0 (February 4, 2020), https://kosovotwopointzero.com/en/bosnia-and-herzegovinas-covid-19-response-threatens-fragile-human-rights/, *archived at* https://perma.cc/Q8Z5-4UXG. See also Jakov Fabinger, "Ethiopian Airlines Flies Huge Boeing 777 to Tiny Bosnian Town," *Simple Flying* (April 24, 2020), https://simpleflying.com/ethiopian-airlines-bosnian-town/, archived at https://perma.cc/47BZ-YMB4 (commenting on the delivery of 200 ventilators to Banja Luka in Republika Srpska as part of an effort to improve the available medical equipment in the entity).

53. See, for example, "COVID-19: Looming Crisis in Developing Countries Threatens to Devastate Economies and Ramp Up Inequality," *United Nations Dev. Program*, https://www.undp.org/content/undp/en/home/news-centre/news/2020/COVID19_Crisis_in_developing_countries_threatens_devastate_economies.html, *archived at* https://perma.cc/BJ9P-GYZJ

54. See, for example, "Comparative Analysis: Definition, Concepts, and Writing Techniques," *Writeawriting* (April 14, 2015), https://www.writeawriting.com/academic-writing/comparative-analysis/

55. Coined in 1883 by the British statistician and social scientist Sir Francis Galton (1822–1911), *eugenics* means "well-born," specifically science "relating to the production of good offspring." See, for example, Charles J. Epstein, "Is Modern Genetics the New Eugenics?" *Genetics in Med.* 5 (2003), 469–75, https://www.nature.com/gim/journal/v5/n6/full/gim2003376a.html (quoting Galton); Ricki Lewis, "Genetic Testing for All: Is it Eugenics?" DNA Science: Genetics in Context (posted September 18, 2014), http://blogs.plos.org/dnascience/2014/09/18/genetic-testing-eugenics/. Both articles appear to suggest that a thin line separates genetic counseling used to minimize transmission of an inherited disorder to offspring and species enhancement. While bearing that fine line in mind, this book limits itself to the narrower meaning.

56. *Gene* or *genome editing* involves "making specific changes to the DNA of a cell or organism" by adding, removing, or altering genetic material at particular locations in the genome, in an attempt to change the characteristics of the cell or organism in question. "What is Genome Editing?" *YourGenome*, https://www.yourgenome.org/facts/what-is-genome-editing, archived at https://perma.cc/7JZ3-TUZV; National Institute of Health, U.S. National Library of Medicine, "What Are Genome Editing and CRISPR-Cas9?" https://ghr.nlm.nih.gov/primer/genomicresearch/genomeediting, archived at https://perma.cc/F4T8-L2VK. One or all of three possibilities could drive such change to the DNA or a cell or organism: for *research* (i.e., to understand the biology of the cell or organism and

how it works); to *treat diseases*, such as leukemia and AIDS; and for *biotech-nology* (i.e., in agriculture to genetically modify crops to improve their yields and resistance to disease and drought). "What is Genome Editing," note 56.

57. See generally Alexandra Minna Stern, *Telling Genes: The Story of Genetic Counseling in America* (Baltimore: Johns Hopkins University Press, 2017).

58. *Bioethics* is the study of the ethical issues emerging from advances in biology and medicine. It is a multidisciplinary field (combining fragments of knowledge from medicine, law, philosophy, public health, public policy, and theology) concerned with the ethical questions that arise in the relationships among life sciences, biotechnology, medicine, politics, law, and philosophy. The field ranges beyond the codes of professional ethics to include attention to social changes brought about by scientific and technological achievements. To the already-difficult question posed by the life sciences as to how far we can go, bioethics adds pertinent queries concerning the relationship between ethics, science, and freedom. UNESCO, "Universal Declaration on Bioethics and Human Rights," *Social and Human Sciences*, http://www.unesco.org/new/en/social-and-human-sciences/themes/bioethics/bioethics-and-human-rights/, archived at https://perma.cc/F8RH-L82M. See also UNESCO, Sector for Social and Human Sciences, *Bioethics Core Curriculum: Section 1: Syllabus Ethics Education Program* (2016), Unit 2, https://unesdoc.unesco.org/ark:/48223/pf0000246885 (discussing "[t]he birth of bioethics") (explaining that Bioethics seeks "to draw attention to the fact that the rapid advances in science ha[ve] proceeded without due attention being paid to values."). More comments on Bioethics can be found in Chap. 8 of this book.

59. Council of Europe, Committee of Ministers, Recommendation No. R (92) 3 on Genetic Testing and Screening for Health Care Purposes (Feb. 10, 1992), Principle 3, *reprinted* in *Int'l Digest of Health Legislation*, 43 (1992), 284, http://hrlibrary.umn.edu/instree/coerecr92-3.html [hereinafter Recommendation No. R (92) 3 on Genetic Testing and Screening for Health Care Purposes]. Founded in 1949, the Council of Europe is an international organization currently made up of 47 member states that is committed to upholding human rights, democracy, and the rule of law in Europe. BiH joined the group in 2002 as 44th member and participates strongly in its affairs. See, for example, Council of Europe, *Action Plan for Bosnia and Herzegovina 2018–2021* (June 13, 2018), https://rm.coe.int/bih-action-plan-2018-2021-en/16808b7563. For explanation of "non-directive" procedure, see Chap. 7.

60. See Sabina Semiz & Philip C. Aka, "Precision Medicine in the Era of CRISPR-Cas9: Evidence from Bosnia and Herzegovina." *Palgrave Communications* (Oct. 2019), https://doi.org/10.1057/s41599-019-0346-2

61. Ibid. ("Challenges of genome editing in the era of CRISPR-Cas9") (commenting on the research scandal involving He Jiankui, a Chinese biophysicist, who disclosed in November of 2018 that he used the CRISPR-Cas9 technique to edit the genes of twin girls reportedly to prevent them from contracting HIV infection).

62. These tests break down into five distinct (sub)categories: diagnostic, predictive (or presymptomatic), carrier, prenatal, and preimplantation. See Orsolya Varga & Jorge Sequeiros, "Definitions of Genetic Testing in European and Other Legal Documents," *EuroGentest*, eurogentest.org/index.php?id=732, archived at https://perma.cc/S6RT-YYUU (appendix); Angela Ballantyne et al., *Medical Genetic Services in Developing Countries: The Ethical, Legal and Social Implications of Genetic Testing and Screening* (WHO, 2006), 15, https://apps.who.int/iris/bitstream/handle/10665/43288/924159344X_eng.pdf?sequence=1&isAllowed=y. *Diagnostic* testing, the most common of these tests, involves the diagnosis of a genetic disease, whether chromosomal or monogenic, in a patient with symptoms. Ballantyne et al., note 62. *Predictive* testing estimates the risk to a person with no symptoms of developing a genetic disease in the future. Varga & Sequeiros, note 62. *Carrier* testing checks whether a healthy individual is a carrier of a recessive mutation that may increase his or her risk of having affected offspring. Ballantyne et al., note 62. *Prenatal* testing, such as for Down Syndrome, identifies a fetus at increased risk of congenital abnormality. Ibid. *Preimplantation* testing, conducted following an in vitro fertilization procedure, is performed on one or two cells removed from the early embryo. Varga & Sequeiros, note 62.

63. Recommendation No. R (92) 3 on Genetic Testing and Screening for Health Care Purposes, note 59, Principle 2 (dealing with quality of genetic services). The applicable guideline here specifies, "[i]t is desirable for centers where laboratory tests are performed to be approved by the State or by a competent authority in the State, and to participate in an external quality assurance." Ibid., p. 2.c.

64. Louiza Kalokairinou, et al. 2018. "Legislation of Direct-to-Consumer Genetic Testing in Europe: A Fragmentary Regulatory Landscape." *J. Community Genet.* 9(2): 117–32 ("Discussion.").

65. See generally ibid.

66. Blatter, note 22.

67. See note 35 and accompanying text.

68. See Roberts et al., note 35, p. 10 (pointing up several methods for evaluating the performance and fairness of a healthcare system that include the WHO's ranking of healthcare systems in the world, assessment based on capacity indicators or on fund flows and payment methods between population groups and institutions, and conceptual frameworks based on economics). For their part, the authors laid out the five "control knobs" of financing, payment, organization, regulation, and behavior for gauging the performance and equity of a healthcare system that they elaborated in their work. See ibid., pp. 153–320.

69. See World Health Organization, *The World Health Report 2000: Health Systems: Improving Performance* (Geneva: World Health Organization, 2000).

# PART I

# Starting Point

# CHAPTER 2

# Background History: Constitutional Law of Healthcare in Bosnia and Herzegovina

**Abstract** This chapter is a historical background account that traces the history of healthcare reforms in Bosnia from socialist Yugoslavia to post-socialist Bosnia. It is a story cast in the constitutional law of healthcare, particularly a commitment to socioeconomic human rights in the land that is sincerely held but lacks deep roots.

**Keywords** Constitutional guarantees for healthcare in socialist Yugoslavia • Constitutional guarantees for healthcare in post-socialist Bosnia

This chapter traces the history of healthcare in Bosnia and Herzegovina. It is a chronological story across two time periods laced in the lingo of socioeconomic human rights, applied in all jurisdictions since the birth of a new independence in 1995, and memorialized in human-right-related instruments, including constitutions and a multilateral treaty. However, although sincerely held, rather than opportunistic, the commitment to socioeconomic human this chapter traces lacks deep root.

© The Author(s) 2020
P. C. Aka, *Genetic Counseling and Preventive Medicine in Post-War Bosnia*, https://doi.org/10.1007/978-981-15-7987-5_2

## CONSTITUTIONAL GUARANTEES FOR HEALTHCARE
## IN SOCIALIST YUGOSLAVIA

After the Second World War (1939–45), Bosnia and Herzegovina became part of former Yugoslavia where, as indicated in Chap. 1, it enjoyed the status of a full republic, one of six autonomous entities under that system.[1] Yugoslavia's 1974 constitution, the most elaborate in the history of the country,[2] contains several more or less specific provisions relating to healthcare. These were, from direct to diffuse, Arts. 186, 162, 163, 192, and 87.

Article 186 stipulated that "[e]very one shall be entitled to *health care*[,]" adding that "cases in which uninsured citizens are entitled to health care from social resources shall be spelled out by statute."[3] Similarly, Art. 162 stipulated that "[w]orkers shall have the right to *health* and other kinds of care and personal security in work."[4] Tied to the right of workers to social security through compulsory social insurance, Art. 163 provided that

> workers shall have, in conformity with statute, the right to *health care* and other benefits in the case of illness, childbirth benefits, benefits in the case of diminution or loss of working capacity, unemployment and old age, and other social security benefits, and for their dependents—the right to *health care*, survivors' pensions, and other social security benefits.[5]

Article 192 stipulated that "[m]an shall have the right to a *healthy* environment. Conditions for realization of this right shall be ensured by the social community."[6] Titled "Conservation and Improvement of the Human Environment," Art. 87 stipulated:

> Working people and citizens [...] shall have the right and duty to assure conditions for the conservation and improvement of the natural and man-made values of the human environment, and to prevent or eliminate harmful consequences of air, soil, water or noise pollution and the like, which endanger these values and imperil the *health* and lives of people.[7]

And, although subject to certain limitations, such as disrupting "the foundation of the socialist self-management democratic order," and endangering the country's independence, among others, these guarantees of healthcare benefits "shall enjoy judicial protection."[8] No less impressive, Yugoslavia ratified the International Covenant on Economic, Social, and Cultural Rights (ICESCR) on June 2, 1971, nearly four years after signing it on August 6, 1967.[9] The ICESCR stipulates, in pertinent part, that state-parties to the treaty "recognize the right of everyone to the enjoyment of the highest attainable standard of physical and mental health."[10] More on this multilateral treaty later in this chapter.

Following the government's assumption of responsibility for healthcare services in 1879 under Austro-Hungarian rule, key events occurred within the healthcare sector in the lead-up to the constitutional provisions recounted above. These include the enactment in 1888 of a law introducing health insurance for some section of the population, introduction of compulsory insurance in 1910 for all employees, and the establishment of the Ministry of Health in 1920.[11] The health ministry was charged with a set of mandates that included healthcare for children, building institutions for preventing and treatment diseases, conducting epidemiological surveillance, and educating the public on healthcare issues.[12] Between 1918 and 1932, the government enacted about 92 health laws.[13]

These key events took place before the onset of socialist rule after the Second World War. Following the advent of the socialist order, the government enacted a law in 1946 that introduced social insurance protection for workers in 1946, extended the protection to children in 1950, and expanded healthcare services within the general population, complete with a corresponding growth in the number of healthcare workers.[14] Industrialization, urbanization, and changes in the social structure of the population in the period from 1961 to 1971 resulted in enhanced specialization of medical personnel and facilities.[15] One indication of this change was the enactment in 1970 of a new law on health insurance and mandatory protection of health.[16] Among other things, the law provided free health services to sections of the population with greater need for medical attention, such as pregnant women, children, and adolescents, while affording protection from certain ill-health conditions, such as infectious diseases, diabetes mellitus, and cancer.[17]

Part of the ideological rivalry that marked the Cold War was a bifurcation of political-civil rights and socioeconomic rights in a division where socialist countries privileged socioeconomic human rights over political-civil human rights and capitalist countries did the opposite.[18] But under Josip B. Tito from 1953 to 1980, Yugoslavia played a "balancing act between East and West, [and] between freedom and authoritarianism."[19] Among other things, particularly for healthcare services, this occurrence suggests that the commitment to socioeconomic human rights was a sincerely held one not actuated by ideological posturing and opportunism.[20]

## CONSTITUTIONAL GUARANTEES FOR HEALTHCARE IN POST-SOCIALIST BOSNIA

In 1993, Bosnia and Herzegovina ratified the ICESCR in its own right as an independent state, free and clear of former Yugoslavia.[21] The treaty codified the provisions in the Universal Declaration of Human Rights (UDHR) on socioeconomic human rights, including the right to healthcare. The UDHR stipulates, in pertinent part, that "[e]very[-]one has the right to a standard of living adequate for the health and well-being of himself and of his family, including food, clothing, housing and medical care."[22] The Universal Declaration is one of numerous human rights instrument that, along with the ICESCR, the Bosnian Constitution of 1995 cites as a source of inspiration,[23] and with respect to the ICESCR, incorporated into the Constitution by reference.[24]

As opposed to a prototypical constitution, the Bosnian Constitution of 1995 was an appendix, Annex 4, to the General Framework Agreement for Peace in Bosnia and Herzegovina which ended the fratricidal war that convulsed the country from 1992 to 1995.[25] It was a culmination of two constitutional experiments by the various entities while the war raged. The first experiment was the constitution of Republika Srpska adopted in 1992, with the aim of creating an independent state tailored only to the interests of Bosnian Serbs.[26] It created a unitary form of government.[27] The second was the Constitution of FBiH, adopted in 1994 as a compromise between Bosniaks and Croats as part of the Washington Agreement. The Constitution established a highly decentralized federation of ten cantons, designed to ensure that Bosniacs and Croats have equal influence on legislation and government, five primarily Bosniac, three primarily Croat, and two cantons of a mixed Bosniac/Croat population.[28]

Next to the two-plus entities that make up BiH, the legal framework for healthcare in FBiH comprises three main instruments: the Constitution, the Law on Health Care,[29] and the Law on Health Insurance.[30] FBiH's Constitution stipulates that "[a]ll persons within the territory of the Federation shall enjoy the right[]" "[t]o health."[31] Between them, the Law on Health Care and the Law on Health Insurance specify the conditions under which persons become eligible to enjoy healthcare benefits, and guarantee each FBiH resident a basic healthcare package, irrespective of income and resources. Specifically, the Law on Health Care governs the principle, organization, and delivery of healthcare services in the Federation, while the Law on Health Insurance regulates health insurance as a part of social insurance, based on certain basic principles like universality, solidarity, and equity.[32] FBiH law guarantees every person the right of equal access to healthcare services,[33] at all three levels of healthcare delivery (primary, secondary, and tertiary),[34] including receipt of medical attention during emergencies.[35] In FBiH, the entity government shares competency for healthcare with the ten cantons.[36] The result is a decentralized arrangement where many responsibilities for healthcare reside with the cantons. There are one Federal Ministry of Health and ten Cantonal Ministries of Health, as well as one Federal Health Insurance and Reinsurance Fund and ten Cantonal Health Insurance Funds.[37] With respect to financing, healthcare in FBiH is predominantly funded from a compulsory stream of contributions commented upon later in Chap. 3 on the characteristic features of BiH healthcare system.[38]

Under RS law, provisions for healthcare parallel those of FBiH in important respects. Here, as in FBiH, the applicable legal framework comprises the Constitution,[39] the Law on Health Care,[40] and the Law on Health Insurance.[41] The Constitution stipulates that "[e]veryone has the right to health care [...] under conditions as provided by law."[42] Although more centralized,[43] like FBiH, RS has similar (but not identical) laws and organizational structures, that perform similar functions. Last but not least, the Statute of the Brčko District, the closest to a constitution for this self-governing unit, includes healthcare among "[t]he functions and powers of the District."[44] Assisted by the Department of Health, the mayor plays an instrumental role in the proposing and implementation of healthcare policies.[45]

This chapter performed the key role ascribed to background histories signified by their ability to start the story of the topic in question, here healthcare reforms, anchored in preventive medicine, from the proverbial beginning, including unearthing activities that shape the current patterns of events.[46] Because awareness "of a country's past" is necessary "to fully understand the nature and issues of its contemporary politics," it is imperative that the researcher look at the politics of a state in question in tandem with "many other activities that have shaped the current pattern of politics."[47] Part of that past history shaping present-day events that, for Bosnia, this chapter unearthed is a commitment to socioeconomic human rights dating back to former Yugoslavia that applies to healthcare. However, although sincerely held, that commitment was not deep-seated. Chapters 3 and 4 indicate why. The first sets forth characteristic features of the Bosnian healthcare system, while the second presents a guide for healthcare reforms in Bosnia made up of four hallmarks, including healthcare as human right.

## NOTES

1. See Chap. 1, note 10, and accompanying text.
2. The document is 304-page long and contains 406 articles. Ustav Socijalisticke Federativne Republike Jugoslvije [Constitution of the Socialist Federal Republic of Yugoslavia] (1974), *translated in* Constitution of the Socialist Federal Republic of Yugoslavia, *World Statesmen.Org*, http://www.worldstatesmen.org/Yugoslavia-Constitution1974.pdf (last visited Mar. 25, 2020).
3. Constitution of the Socialist Federal Republic of Yugoslavia (1974), Art. 186 (emphasis added).
4. Ibid., Art. 162 (emphasis added).
5. Ibid., Art. 163 (emphasis added).
6. Ibid., Art. 192 (emphasis added).
7. Ibid., Art. 87 (emphasis added).
8. Ibid., Art. 203.
9. "Chapter IV – Human Rights: 3. International Covenant on Economic, Social and Cultural Rights," *United Nations Treaty Collection*, https://treaties.un.org/Pages/ViewDetails.aspx?src=IND&mtdsg_no=IV-3&chapter=4&lang=en, archived at https://perma.cc/N22X-CNMY [hereinafter "Chapter IV—Human Rights"] (End-Note 3). The difference between signature and ratification is that, although, unlike ratification, signature establishes no consent to be bound, at the same time it creates an obligation to "refrain from acts that would defeat or undermine" the objective or purpose of the treaty. See Vienna Convention on the Law of Treaties Art. 18, *opened for signature* May 23, 1969, 1115 U.N.T.S. 331, Art.18.
10. ICESCR, U.N. Gen. Assembly Resolution No. 2200A (XXI) (December 16, 1966, entered into force on January 3, 1976), Art. 12(1). The treaty goes so far as to lay out measures that these state-parties could use to realize consummation of this right for their citizens. These include reduction of the stillbirth rate and of infant mortality, and the healthy development of the child; improving all aspects of environmental and industrial hygiene; combatting all diseases, epidemic, endemic, and occupational; and creating

conditions designed to guarantee medical service and attention to all their citizens in the event of sickness. Ibid., Art. 12(2)(a)-(d).

11. Jennifer Cain et al., eds. *Health Care Systems in Transition: Bosnia and Herzegovina* (Copenhagen: European Observatory on Health Care Systems, 2002), 14.

12. Ibid., p. 15.

13. Ibid.

14. Ibid., p. 16.

15. Ibid.

16. Ibid.

17. Ibid.

18. See Philip C Aka, "Fidel Castro and Socioeconomic Human Rights in Africa: A Multi-Level Analysis," *Fordham Int'l L. J.* 43 (Fall 2019), 73.

19. Jason Farago, "When Yugoslavia's Bright Future Was Fashioned in Concrete," *Wral* (July 19, 2018), https://www.wral.com/when-yugoslavia-s-bright-future-was-fashioned-in-concrete/17708739/

20. As explained elsewhere with respect to Cuba under Fidel Castro, but equally true of many other socialist states, the bifurcation never made sense in that economic, social, and cultural or socioeconomic human rights are guarantees of freedom that, in addition to affordable healthcare, encompass access to nutritious food, livable shelter, affordable and skill-rich education, to enable individuals to provide these goods for themselves, without which non-socioeconomic rights, including even the right to life, ring hollow. See Aka, note 18, pp. 49–50.

21. "Chapter IV—Human Rights," note 9; see also Constitution of Bosnia and Herzegovina, Annex 4 to the General Framework Agreement for Peace in Bosnia and Herzegovina (more popularly known as the Dayton Agreement). Constitution of Bosnia and Herzegovina (1995), pmbl., http://www.ohr.int/ohr-dept/legal/laws-of-bih/pdf/001%20-%20 Constitutions/BH/BH%20CONSTITUTION%20.pdf (unpublished version of the document) (acknowledging the inspiration of the ICESCR and other human rights instruments); ibid., Annex 1 (listing the ICESCR as No. 8 among "additional human rights agreements to be applied in Bosnia and Herzegovina.").

22. Universal Declaration of Human Rights, U.N. General Assembly Resolution No. 217A (December 10, 1948), Art. 25(1).

23. See Constitution of Bosnia and Herzegovina, note 21, pmbl.

24. Constitution of Bosnia and Herzegovina, note 21, Annex 1 (listing the ICESCR as No. 8 among "additional human rights agreements to be applied in Bosnia and Herzegovina.").

25. See Constitution of Bosnia and Herzegovina, note 21. The document comprises twelve articles, plus a preamble, dealing with multiple issues,

including human rights and fundamental freedoms (Art. 2), responsibilities of the central and entity governments and relationship between these organs (Art. 3), legislative institutions and powers (Art. 4), executive institutions and powers (Art. 5), judicial institutions, particularly the Constitutional Court, and powers (Art. 6), monetary institutions, particularly the Central Bank, and powers (Art. 7), and finances (Art. 8), among others. Ibid. The other annexes to the peace agreement, eleven of them altogether, are the following: Agreement on Military Aspects of the Peace Settlement (Annex 1-A), Agreement on Regional Stabilization (Annex 1-B), Agreement on Inter-Entity Boundary Line and Related Issues (Annex 2), Agreement on Elections (Annex 3), Agreement on Arbitration (Annex 5), Agreement on Human Rights (Annex 6), Agreement on Refugees and Displaced Persons (Annex 7), Agreement on the Commission to Preserve National Monuments (Annex 8), Agreement on Bosnia and Herzegovina Public Corporations (Annex 9), Agreement on Civilian Implementation (Annex 10), and Agreement on International Police Task Force (Annex 11). See General Framework Agreement for Peace in Bosnia and Herzegovina, accessible at: https://www.osce.org/bih/126173?download=true. The warring parties who reached this agreement were: BiH, Croatia, and Yugoslavia. Eight signatories to the agreement were Slobodan Milošević for Bosnian Serbs, Alija Izetbegović for BiH, Franjo Tuđman for Croatia, Bill Clinton for the United States, Jacques Chirac for France, John Major for the United Kingdom, Helmut Kohl for Germany, and Victor Chernomyrdin for Russia. The agreement was witnessed by the United States, France, the United Kingdom, Germany, Russia, and the European Union. See Summary of the Dayton Peace Agreement on Bosnia and Herzegovina, University of Minnesota Hum. Rts. Library (November 30, 1995), http://hrlibrary.umn.edu/icty/dayton/daytonsum.html

26. Azra Branković, "Administrative Structure of Bosnia and Herzegovina," *in* Yucel Oğurlu & Ahmed Mulanić, eds, *Bosnia and Herzegovina: Law, Society[,] and Politics* (Sarajevo: Int'l Univ. of Sarajevo, 2016), 23.

27. Council of Europe, *The Honoring of Obligations and Commitment by Bosnia and Herzegovina*, Doc. No. 14465 (Parliamentary Assembly, January 8, 2019), 8, ¶ 19.

28. Branković, note 26, p. 23.

29. Law on Health Care, FBiH, Official Gazette of the Federation of Bosnia and Herzegovina, 46/10, and 75/13.

30. Law on Health Insurance, FBiH, Official Gazette of the Federation of Bosnia and Herzegovina, 30/97, 7/02, 70/08, and 48/11.

31. See Constitution of the Federation of Bosnia and Herzegovina (1994), Official Gazette of the Federation of Bosnia and Herzegovina, 1/94,

https://advokat-prnjavorac.com/legislation/constitution_fbih.pdf,
Art. 2(o).

32. Marko Martić & Ognjen Đukić, Friedrich Ebert Stiftung Sarajevo, "Health
Care Systems in BiH: Financing Challenges and Reform Options?"
(October 2017), 5, https://library.fes.de/pdf-files/bueros/sara-
jevo/14124.pdf. *Universality* is present when no one is denied access to
healthcare; *solidarity* is linked to the need to ensure accessibility to all; and
*equity* relates to equal access according to need, without regard to gender,
age, social status, or ability to pay. Ibid.

33. Law on Health Care, FBIH, note 29, Art. 26.

34. See United Nations High Commissioner for Refugees' Office of the Chief
of Mission in Bosnia, *Health Care in Bosnia and Herzegovina in the Context
of the Return of Refugees and Displaced Persons* (Sarajevo: July 2001), 25–7
[hereinafter *Health Care in BiH*]. Elsewhere, this UNCHR source denom-
inated them primary, specialist-consulting, and hospital. See ibid., p. 16.
This book sticks with the less complex primary-secondary-tertiary
classification.

35. For more, see Chap. 3 (analyzing the features of the Bosnian healthcare
system).

36. Constitution of FBiH, note 31, Art. III (2,b), in conjunction with Art. II.

37. See Martić & Đukić, note 32, p. 6, including Chart 1, displaying the organizational structure of the healthcare system in FBiH.

38. Martić & Đukić, note 32, p. 7.

39. See generally Constitution of Republika Srpska, Official Gazette of
Republika Srpska No. 2/92, https://advokat-prnjavorac.com/legisla-
tion/Constitution-of-Republika-Srpska.pdf

40. Law on Health Care, Republika Srpska Official Gazette No. 18/99,
Art. 10.

41. Law on Health Insurance, Republika Srpska Official Gazette No. 18/99.

42. Constitution of Republika Srpska, note 39, Art. 37. More precisely, the
Constitution provides that "[c]hildren, pregnant women and elderly persons shall be entitled to health care financed out of the public funds, while
other persons shall enjoy such a care under the conditions spelled out in a
law." Ibid.

43. The political entity has seven regions, but with nothing close to the autonomy of the cantons in FBiH: Banja Luka (putative capital), Doboj, Bijeljina,
Vlasenica, Sarajevo-Romanija or Sokolac, Foča, and Trebinje.

44. Statute of the Brčko District of Bosnia and Herzegovina (2000), https://
advokat-prnjavorac.com/legislation/Statute-of-the-Brcko-Distrikt-of-
Bosnia-and-Herzegovina.pdf, Art. 8, item (g), "Health Care."

45. See, for example, ibid., Art. 52(2) (giving the mayor responsibility for
implementing the laws of BiH as well as of the District); ibid., Art. 52(3)

(making the mayor responsible to the District Assembly for the "orderly management and administration of the District.").

46. See Frank L. Wilson, *Concepts and Issues in Comparative Politics: An Introduction* (Upper Saddle River, N.J.: Prentice Hall, 1996), 17.

47. Ibid.

# CHAPTER 3

# Features of the Bosnian Healthcare System

**Abstract**  This chapter describes the characteristic features of the Bosnian healthcare system, including the three levels of healthcare delivery in the country. The discussion anticipates the assessment of the healthcare system undertaken in Chap. 4.

**Keywords**  Health • Healthcare system • Bismarck model of healthcare • Health Insurance Fund • Three levels of Bosnian healthcare delivery • Four channels of primary healthcare in Bosnia • *Bolnica* (secondary healthcare) • *Klinicki Centar* (Clinical Centers) (tertiary healthcare)

This chapter analyzes the features of Bosnian healthcare system. There are two aspects to the discussion in this chapter: presentation of the two characteristic features of the Bosnian healthcare system, and a delineation of the three levels of healthcare delivery and services.

## Defining a Healthcare System

*Health* is "[t]he capacity to live a full, active[,] and breathing life[,]" and a property that ranks "among the most precious treasures" humans have.[1] Building on this proposition, a *healthcare system* consists of any assemblage of people and things, including funding and information technology, of varying degree of integration or organizational management, whose

© The Author(s) 2020
P. C. Aka, *Genetic Counseling and Preventive Medicine in Post-War Bosnia*, https://doi.org/10.1007/978-981-15-7987-5_3

primary intent is to promote, restore, or maintain health.[2] This composite includes formal health services like the delivery of personal medical attention by a doctor, whether dispenser of orthodox or traditional medicine; taking care of the sick at home; activities designed to promote health and prevent diseases; and interventions designed to improve health, such as road safety and environmental safety campaigns.[3]

It is not all. Instead, the definition equally encompasses activities outside this formal boundaries ultimately tied to health like increased school enrollment for girls and changing the educational curriculum to make students better future caregivers and consumers of healthcare.[4] Multiple features which influence a country's healthcare system include the unique culture and history of the society, priorities given to certain ethical values (such as autonomy of patients and healthcare providers), and the level of economic resources available for healthcare.[5]

## Two Characteristic Features of Bosnia's Healthcare System

The first feature of the BiH healthcare system is its fragmentation into numerous small units. Compared to the unified structure in former Yugoslavia,[6] the BiH healthcare system is fragmented into thirteen units: FBiH, its ten Cantons, RS, and Brčko District.[7] The fragmentation complicates the provision of healthcare services, "increases management and coordination costs and adversely affects the rationality of management of healthcare institutions, primarily through the prism of untapped opportunities of economy of scope."[8]

The second, far more elaborate, characteristic feature is the "Bismarck [m]odel" of healthcare, whereby access to healthcare services is provided through mandatory health insurance, based on deductions from workers' salaries and other more or less related sources, rather than from government budgets.[9] Consistent with the model, each of the thirteen units that, collectively, comprise the Bosnian healthcare system offers two types of health insurance: *compulsory*, which covers most citizens; and *extended*, a private, voluntary scheme for citizens who desire more coverage beyond the level provided by the conventional method.[10] Because most citizens are covered under the first category, the ensuing discussion focuses mainly on that compulsory category. Under the compulsory scheme, the residents who receive employment income make contributions, which are deducted from their salaries and paid as follows: (a) for employed persons, by their employer; (b) for pensioners, by the relevant pension fund; (c) for persons dependent on social welfare, by the relevant welfare institution; and (d) for unemployed persons, by the Employment Bureau that they are registered with.[11] These monies are then paid to the appropriate governmental entity or sub-entity (e.g., cantonal), which is then responsible for providing healthcare services to residents within its area of authority.[12]

Insured persons, individuals with health insurance who are obligated to make contributions to receive healthcare benefits, form a key element of the compulsory system. Based on the level of insurance coverage, these individuals may be divided into several categories: directly insured; insurance holders, such as family members, who are insured through the insured person, for whom no contribution is made; persons insured solely for "occupational diseases and work-related injuries; and foreign nationals insured [based] on [. . .] signed bilateral agreements."[13] Using Republika Srpska from 2014 to 2018 as a case in point, Table 3.1 depicts the structure of insured persons, together with their respective shares in the total revenue of the Health Insurance Fund. Table 3.1 highlights four notable facts. First, employees represent 35% of insured persons, but contribute almost 84% to the total revenue. Second, pensioners comprise more than 33% of insured persons but contribute a miniscule 2.9% to the total revenue. To put things into perspective, in RS, pensioners' contribution is a marked departure from the figures of neighboring countries like Serbia

**Table 3.1** Structure of insured persons and their shares in the total revenue of the RS Health Insurance Fund (numbers in rounded percentages)

| Item No. | Insured category | Share in total number of the insured (%) | Share in total revenue (%) |
|---|---|---|---|
| 1. | Employees | 35 | 84 |
| 2. | Pensioners | 33 | 3 |
| 3. | Farmers | 0.4 | 0.3 |
| 4. | Unemployed persons | 25 | 7 |
| 5. | Disabled persons from the war | 0.8 | 0.1 |
| 6. | Refugees and displaced persons | 0.1 | 0.1 |
| 7. | Foreign insured persons | 5 | 5 |
| 8. | Social Work Center | 0.4 | 0.4 |

Martić and Đukić, note 7, p. 19, citing the Strategic Plan of the RS Health Insurance Fund, 2014–2018

(24%), North Macedonia (approximately 22%), Montenegro (approximately 20%), and Slovenia (approximately 17%).[14] Together, employees and pensioners contribute nearly 87% to the total revenue of the Health Insurance Fund. Third, as a group, foreign workers comprise little over 5% of the general population, but generate nearly 5% of the total revenue in a share that mimics their share of the population. Joined to employees and pensioners, collectively, these three groups contribute 92% of the total revenue necessary to maintain the healthcare system. Finally, unemployed persons who represent nearly 25% of the population of insured persons (one out of every four insured persons) contribute little over 7% of share to the total revenue of the Health Insurance Fund—as indicated in the previous paragraph, paid for them by the employment agency they are registered with.

Under the compulsory scheme, only insured persons are entitled to healthcare. Persons without insurance must make out-of-pocket payments to healthcare providers at the time of service, except during emergencies.[15] Under Bosnian healthcare laws, medical assistance must be "provided to all persons in cases of emergency, regardless of ability to pay";[16] as such, physicians who fail to provide emergency aid may face criminal sanctions.[17] These emergency situations include "assistance with [childbirth] outside of hospitals, emergency transportation of sick and injured persons and women in labor to appropriate health institutions, medical treatment of sick and injured persons in health institutions or at home during weekends and holidays, [and] resuscitation during transportation."[18]

In return for their contributions, insured persons receive a variety of services that, in addition to regular healthcare services, include sick leave pay, reimbursement for healthcare-related travel costs, and any other entitlements established by the applicable Health Insurance Fund of the unit in question.[19] Family members can also be reimbursed for healthcare-related travel expenses, including treatment of work-related injuries and illnesses, treatment of drug addiction, and provision of blood bank services.[20] To access services in any BiH entity, insured persons must register and apply for a certified health insurance card.[21] For validation purposes, the branch office of the applicable Health Insurance Fund generally certifies cards monthly; children's and farmers' cards, however, may be certified quarterly.[22] In all jurisdictions, those over fifteen years of age who are not in school can obtain personal health insurance by registering with the Employment Bureau.[23] Unemployed persons must also register with Employment Bureaus to gain access to health insurance and healthcare.[24]

To receive treatment, insured persons must pay a fixed copay, called "participat[ory] fee," that is determined by the applicable Health Insurance Fund.[25] However, in many jurisdictions, the following individuals may be exempted from these copays: pregnant women, those with a baby less than one-year old, children under fifteen, senior citizens (i.e., persons sixty-five and above), handicapped persons, persons with certain contagious diseases, and persons with psychiatric and neuromuscular diseases.[26]

RS, unlike FBiH, has centralized healthcare services via the Ministry of Health and Social Welfare of Republika Srpska, the Health Insurance Fund of Republika Srpska, and the Public Health Institute of Republika Srpska.[27] The RS Ministry of Health and Social Welfare coordinates healthcare activities, "creates business policies and development strategies, [and] plans and coordinates the work of the health institutions network," among other responsibilities.[28] Along with other health institutions, the Health Insurance Fund of RS delivers primary, secondary, and tertiary healthcare services.[29] There are about 364 other health institutions listed in the Health Institution Register with the Ministry of Health and Social Welfare of RS.[30] Last but not least, the Public Health Institute of RS conducts research and education relating to public health and monitors RS residents' health.[31] Like in FBiH, the Health Insurance Fund of RS's main income sources include contributions for health insurance deducted from workers' salaries, contributions by pension beneficiaries, contributions from farmers, and contributions for the unemployed and other categories (made for them by the government).[32]

In Brčko District, however, responsibility for enforcing laws and regulations relating to healthcare falls on the mayor, who is assisted by the Department of Health.[33] This is true at all three applicable levels: primary, secondary, and (partially) tertiary.[34] But, like in the two entities, FBiH and RS, healthcare financing occurs through a Health Insurance Fund, primarily based on contributions from workers, farmers, and persons who are retired, self-employed, and unemployed, among other categories.[35] The Assembly of Brčko District, the closest entity to a legislature in this self-governing unit, decides the base and rate of contribution to the Health Insurance Fund.[36]

Contrary to the suggestion of inclusiveness that it connotes, the compulsory system still leaves many individuals and groups uncovered.[37] These uncovered individuals include workers whose years of service have not been "linked," self-employed persons who for any reason failed to pay their health insurance contributions, and unemployed persons who failed to extend their registration with the applicable employment agencies.[38] Overall, more than 15% of the BiH population is not covered.[39] For example, from 2008 to 2015, FBiH covered about 85% of its population, while RS covered about 70%.[40] Some analysts speculate that this disparity results because "a higher share of [the] population [is] engaged in agriculture" in RS, a group that is often left out of the compulsory contribution framework.[41]

However, examined more closely, the higher coverage in FBiH is not as impressive as it looks at first sight because there are significant differences in coverage among the cantons in FBiH (see Table 3.2). Among FBiH cantons, large variations exist in employment rates and salary levels, which are two variables that are used to compute healthcare contributions.[42] Based on information presented in Table 3.2, from 2010 to 2015, Sarajevo Canton and Western-Herzegovina Canton registered an average of 95% coverage, whereas Canton 10, for example, registered an average of approximately 66%. The model of healthcare financing in the cantons, which are based mainly on employee contributions, engenders inequality among insured persons, "depending on the economic position of the canton and the place where the insured persons live."[43] In practical terms, this means cantons with fewer employees and lower salaries will have "lower health insurance coverage and lower allocations for public healthcare services per insured person."[44] However, citizens living in "poorer" cantons

**Table 3.2**   Health insurance coverage in FBiH by Cantons, 2010–2015 (in rounded percentages)

| Year | 2010 | 2011 | 2012 | 2013 | 2014 | 2015 |
| --- | --- | --- | --- | --- | --- | --- |
| Una-Sana | 73 | 73 | 74 | 74 | 73 | 72 |
| Posavina | 79 | 79 | 79 | 77 | 76 | 75 |
| Tuzla | 88 | 88 | 89 | 90 | 89 | 88 |
| Zenica-Doboj | 82 | 86 | 87 | 87 | 87 | 86 |
| Bosnian-Podrinje | 78 | 78 | 79 | 81 | 79 | 79 |
| Central Bosnia | 84 | 85 | 87 | 85 | 86 | 86 |
| Herzegovina-Neretva | 84 | 84 | 85 | 85 | 86 | 87 |
| West Herzegovina | 90 | 92 | 92 | 97 | 100 | 97 |
| Sarajevo | 94 | 94 | 96 | 95 | 95 | 96 |
| Canton 10 | 67 | 67 | 67 | 64 | 64 | 64 |

Martić & Đukić, note 7, p. 9, tbl. 2 (citing Federal Insurance and Reinsurance Fund)

have no less need for health insurance than their counterparts in more affluent cantons.[45]

The gaps in coverage between FBiH and RS, and among the Cantons in FBiH, smack of discrimination, which is inconsistent with equity and equality in healthcare studies.[46] Those gaps imply that certain categories of the population, such as individuals who reside in rural areas, the poor, Romas, and uneducated persons, lack coverage, meaning they will seek to satisfy their healthcare needs in the commercial private sector, use quack doctors, or forego healthcare services altogether.[47] Attempts to address this issue in places like FBiH, where the government set up a Solidarity Fund, have not been successful, largely because those interventions fell short of redefining the structure of healthcare funding.[48]

## THREE LEVELS IN BOSNIAN HEALTHCARE

One element of the Bosnian healthcare system complementary to the two features analyzed in the previous section, yet distinct enough to warrant separate treatment are the three levels of healthcare delivery and services in the land. The three levels are primary, secondary, and tertiary. The thirteen units (organized around two entities) that form this system emphasize these three levels to various degrees.[49] Primary healthcare forms the bulk of the healthcare system. In BiH, primary healthcare is designed to cover 70–80% of all medical cases (even though in reality it covers only 10–20%). This care level is dispensed through four channels: *Ambulanta* (AMB),[50] Domovi zdravlja (DZ, or "house of health"),[51] Hitna pomoci (HP, or first aid and emergency medicine),[52] and Farmacia (PH, or pharmacy).[53]

AMBs are basic ambulatory primary healthcare found in practically every village. In this primary setting, usually a nurse does the daily work, with a general practitioner often visiting once or more a week, except in larger villages, where the general practitioner visits every day. In AMBs, both the services rendered and the equipment used to provide those services are basic and minimal. AMB services include anamnesis,[54] clinical checks (e.g., noninvasive blood pressure, pulse rate, and temperature), prescription of few drugs, and patient referrals to a DZ. AMB's equipment includes basic items like a Riva-Rocci,[55] stethoscope, and thermometer.

DZs are a second channel through which primary healthcare is dispensed in BiH. DZs are advanced ambulatory healthcare institutions located in the main villages of each municipality. DZs usually function in tandem with first aid or emergency medicine (HP) and sometimes connect to a pharmacy (PH). This pharmaceutical connection is significant, considering that in BiH, AMBs hardly refer patients directly to a hospital. Medical services at DZs include labs with facilities, such as ultrasound, endoscopy, and advanced X-ray machines. However, the use of such equipment, especially sophisticated ones, depends on availability of specialists and items like films, probes, and ultrasound gel. Staff who operate such equipment include general practitioners, epidemiologists, occupational therapists, gynecologists, obstetricians, and pediatricians.

At DZs, an array of specialists from public hospitals or in private practice (on special contracts with the government) visits DZs once or twice per week or month. These specialists include radiologists, experts in infectious disease, experts in internal medicine, ophthalmologists, experts in enterology, neuropsychiatrists, pneumo-physiologists, and orthopedic doctors, if available. Occasionally, these specialists include experts on family medicine and emergency medicine, but such specialists mostly work at the higher HP level. In Bosnia, access to specialist services, where these attentions are available, sometimes are based not on medical need but extra-medical factors, such as political connections.

The third channel used to dispense primary healthcare in BiH is HP. HPs are an amalgam of first aid center, emergency room, and transport center. HPs are usually located in a DZ and operate twenty-four hours a day and seven days a week. In large cities, such as Sarajevo, HPs have their own independent building and infrastructure. Patients can access the services of an HP either directly or via phone call. In theory, "[n]ormally a car or ambulance is sent and[,] if available[,] a nurse, medical technician, and/or doctor will be sent as well."[56] In actual practice, ambulances are minimally equipped and sometimes, at best, are outfitted with oxygen (i.e., ventilators). In other words, few HPs have well-equipped emergency cars or ambulances; HPs' work tools are often donated. If and when a doctor accompanies these vehicles, the doctor usually carries basic medicinal materials.

Farmacia (PH) are the fourth channel used to dispense primary healthcare in Bosnia. This channel comprises pharmacies run by the government, private pharmacies, and a scatter of humanitarian pharmacies stocked with drugs donated by international humanitarian organizations. Although there are also free-standing ones, many state pharmacies are separate, and many are attached to DZs where they support local healthcare facilities and provide basic drug materials to patients, such as bandages, syringes, and vials. Pharmacies operated by international humanitarian organizations are also associated with DZs and sometimes with General Hospitals as well.

Secondary healthcare is provided mainly in general hospitals (Bolnica), usually located in the capitals of each canton (in the case of the FBiH). Tertiary care is provided mainly at Clinical Centers (CC, or *Klinicki Centar* in Bosnian language). These healthcare institutions are often affiliated to tertiary institutions like universities and are generally located in capitals and other major cities, such as Sarajevo, Tuzla, and Mostar in FBiH, and Luka and Foca/Srbinje in RS. They are at the apex of the healthcare pecking order imbued with the capacity to provide healthcare of the highest scope in every specialty along with the necessary equipment to render those services.[57] In principle, they are health institutions of last resort in referral "when GHs are not in a position to provide the necessary expertise, diagnosis, or treatment."[58]

Although necessary, focus on the features of BiH healthcare system by itself is insufficient, unless accompanied by complementing examination regarding the extent to which those features meet the healthcare needs of citizens today. Put differently, because of the problems with the Bosnian healthcare system this chapter unearths, especially the first section pertaining to the features of the system, this chapter is a down-payment on the critical assessment of the system Chap. 4, next after this, undertakes.

## NOTES

1. Paola Testori Coggi, "Foreword from the European Commission," *in* Irene Papanicolas & Peter C. Smith, *Health System Performance Comparison: An Agenda for Policy Information and Research* (Maidenhead, UK: Open University Press, 2013), xi.

2. World Health Organization, *The World Health Report 2000: Health Systems: Improving Performance* (Geneva: World Health Organization, 2000), 1, 5; Mary Ko Zimmerman, "Comparative Health-Care Systems," *Encyclopedia of Sociology* (updated Jan. 25, 2020), https://www.encyclopedia.com/social-sciences/encyclopedias-almanacs-transcripts-and-maps/comparative-health-care-systems. See also I. Gregory Pawlson et al., "Healthcare Systems," *Encyclopedia of Bioethics* (updated Dec. 4, 2019), https://www.encyclopedia.com/science/encyclopedias-almanacs-transcripts-and-maps/healthcare-systems (stating that "[t]he goal of a healthcare system is to enhance the health of the population in the most effective manner possible in light of a society's available resources and competing needs.").

3. *World Health Report 2000*, note 2, p. 5.
4. Ibid. See also Marina Karanikolos et al., "Comparing Population Health," *in* Irene Papanicolas & Peter C. Smith, *Health System Performance Comparison: An Agenda for Policy Information and Research* (Maidenhead, UK: Open University Press, 2013), 128.
5. Pawlson et al., note 2.
6. See United Nations High Commissioner for Refugees' Office of the Chief of Mission in Bosnia, *Health Care in Bosnia and Herzegovina in the Context of the Return of Refugees and Displaced Persons* (Sarajevo: July 2001) [hereinafter *Health Care in BiH*], p. i (Executive Summary), p. 1 (introduction).
7. Marko Martić & Ognjen Đukić, Friedrich Ebert Stiftung Sarajevo, "Health Care Systems in BiH: Financing Challenges and Reform Options?" (October 2017), 6, https://library.fes.de/pdf-files/bueros/sarajevo/14124.pdf. Instructively, in their piece referenced repeatedly in this research, Martić and Đukić used the plural healthcare system*s*, rather than the singular.
8. Martić & Đukić, note 7, p. 6.
9. See generally Martić & Đukić, 7. The Bismarck model harks back to German Chancellor Otto von Bismarck (1815–1898), whose introduction of a statutory health insurance in 1883 in Germany paved the way for a comprehensive social insurance system. Bismarck's goal was twofold: counter social unrest and socialism, as well as weaken economically the voluntary social insurance of the trade unions and church-run labor federations. "Bismarck versus Beveridge: A Comparison of Social Insurance Systems in Europe," *Cesifo Dice Rept.* (April 2008), 69–70, https://www.ifo.de/DocDL/dicereport408-db6.pdf
10. *Health Care in BiH*, note 6, p. 2; Bosnia and Herzegovina, Third Report of BiH on Implementation of the European Social Charter [Revised] (Nov. 2012), http://www.mhrr.gov.ba/PDF/LjudskaPrava/III%20IZVJESTAJ%20GRUPA%202%20eng.pdf ("[For example,] [t]he Law on Health Insurance [in Republika Srpska] governs the system of mandatory and extended health insurance, insurance rights, [and] the exercise of rights and principles of private health insurance."). See also Osman Slipicević & Adisa Malicbegović, "Public and Private Sector[s] in the Health Care System of the Federation [of] Bosnia and Herzegovina: Policy and Strategy," *Materia Socio Medica* [*J. of Acad. Of Med. Sciences of Bosn. & Herz.*], 24(1) (2012), 54–7, doi https://doi.org/10.5455/msm.2012.24.54-57, ncbi.nlm.nih.gov/pmc/articles/PMC3633389/
11. See *Health Care in BiH*, note 6, p. 15 (relating to RS).
12. Ibid., p. 2.
13. Martić & Đukić, note 7, p. 8.

14. Ibid., p. 20 (quoting figures for 2011).
15. *Health Care in BiH*, note 6, p. 14.
16. Ibid., p. 7 & n.45, citing The Law on Health Care, Art. 39 (Official Gazette of Republika Srpska, No. 18/99) (mandating the organization of healthcare such that emergency medical assistance, including transportation, is available at any time).
17. See *Health Care in BiH*, note 6, p. 7, n. 45, citing FBiH Criminal Code, art. 246; and RS Criminal Code, Art. 204.
18. *Health Care in BiH,* note 6, p. 19.
19. Ibid., pp. 3–4, 3 n.19, citing The Law on Health Insurance, Art. 31 (Official Gazette of the Federation of Bosnia and Herzegovina, No. 30/97, 7/02, 70/08, and 48/11) and The Law of Health Insurance, Arts. 18–19 (Official Gazette of Republika Srpska, No. 18/99).
20. Ibid., pp. 18, 18 n.102, citing The Law of Health Insurance, Art. 32 (Official Gazette of the Federation of Bosnia and Herzegovina, No. 30/97, 7/02, 70/08, and 48/11).
21. Martić & Đukić, note 7, p. 8.
22. Ibid.
23. Ibid.
24. Ibid.
25. See ibid., p. 7.
26. "Medicine in Bosnia-Herzegovina," *Best Country*, http://www.best-country.com/europe/bosnia_herzegovina/medicine, *archived at* https://perma.cc/758U-J5DJ; The Law of Health Insurance, arts. 44–45 (Official Gazette of the Federation of Bosnia and Herzegovina, No. 30/97, 7/02, 70/08, and 48/11).
27. Ibid., p. 7.
28. Ibid.
29. *Health Care in BiH*, note 6, pp. 25–7 (covering RS alongside FBiH).
30. Martić & Đukić, note 7, p. 8.
31. Ibid., pp. 7–8.
32. Ibid., p. 8.
33. Martić & Đukić, note 7, p. 8. This structure of responsibility is consistent with the Statute of the District (its constitutional document) and the Health Insurance Law of Brčko District. Ibid.
34. Ibid.
35. Martić & Đukić, note 7, p. 8.
36. See ibid., citing Decision on the Base and Rate of Contribution for Health Insurance (Official Gazette of the Brčko District of BiH, 37/2009).
37. *Health Care in BiH*, note 6, p. 1 ("[W]hile the vast majority of the BiH population is nominally covered by a public compulsory health insurance

scheme, in practi[c]e[,] many BiH residents experience difficulty in accessing health care."). See also Martić & Đukić, note 7, p. 8.

38. Ibid., p. 8, n. 6.
39. Ibid., p. 8.
40. Ibid., p. 8, 9 tbl. 1 (including the methodological explanation under the table justifying the assessment of about 70% coverage for RS)
41. Ibid., p. 8.
42. Martić & Đukić, note 7, p. 27.
43. Ibid., p. 15.
44. Ibid.
45. Ibid.
46. See Martić & Đukić, note 7, p. 9.
47. See ibid. Romani people are the largest of the seventeen national minority groups that Bosnian law recognizes. More than other groups, majority or minority, the Romani people "suffer from poverty, discrimination[,] and social exclusion from childhood onward." *See* Hoi Mun Yee, "Bosnia's Roma Try to Break Out of Isolation, *BalkanInsight* (June 14, 2017), https://balkaninsight.com/2017/06/14/bosnia-s-roma-try-to-break-out-of-isolation-06-13-2017-2/
48. Martić & Đukić, note 7, p. 15. See also ibid., p. 25 (enumerating "[c]urrent initiatives for reform of health financing schemes" in the country). One of these suggestions for reform include the initiative by Jasmin Imamović, Mayor of Tuzla, who advocated rationalization of the healthcare system in FBiH by abolishing the system of healthcare management at the cantonal level and transferring competencies to the entity and local levels. Ibid., p. 25. However, the proposal triggered "different political reactions in FBiH and […] there is still no unanimous political opinion on the matter nor the willingness to implement the solutions" the initiative signifies. Ibid., p. 26.
49. This section draws from *Health Care in BiH*, note 6, pp. 25–7.
50. *Ambulanta* is Slovak for *infirmary.*
51. Dom zdravlje (DZ) equates to "House of Health" in Croatian language.
52. Hitna pomoc (HP) is Bosnian for *ambulance.*
53. Farmacia is Italian for *pharmacy.*
54. The term means a tale of medical history told by the patient himself or herself, especially at the beginning of the doctor–patient relationship.
55. This term refers to a devise used to measure blood pressure.
56. *Health Care in BiH*, note 7, p. 26.
57. Ibid.
58. Ibid., p. 27.

# PART II

# Healthcare Reforms as Human Rights in Bosnia

# Four Hallmarks of a Good Healthcare System: A Guide for Healthcare Reforms in Bosnia

**Abstract** This chapter lays out four hallmarks of a good healthcare system—good laws, adequate financing, healthcare as human rights, and good politics—presented as a guide for healthcare reforms in Bosnia, together with an assessment of the Bosnian healthcare system's performance on each of the hallmarks.

**Keywords** Four hallmarks of a good healthcare system • Responsiveness in healthcare

This chapter sets forth the hallmarks of a good healthcare system, laid out in this book as a guide for healthcare reforms in Bosnia. The discussion integrates an assessment of the Bosnian healthcare system's performance on each of the hallmarks. The material builds on, complements, and enriches the discussion in Chap. 3 on the general features of the BiH healthcare system, including a statement on the three levels of healthcare delivery and services. Performance is intrinsic to the vitality of a healthcare system. It is a variable, in turn, based on yardsticks that form the basis for meaningful assessment and analysis.

Different studies use different measures for gauging the performance of a healthcare system.[1] The set of measures used here is a simplified yardstick that mimics methods in the literature, but departs from those methods in terms of its increased accent on human rights. This is an orientation inherent in the definition of healthcare that slowly but steadily is gaining traction in some section of the literature.[2] The measures also build on the assessment instrument—made up of health level and distribution, responsiveness level and distribution, fairness in financial contributions, health expenditure per capita, and level of health performance—that the World Health Organization introduced in its seminal report in 2000.[3] As a measurement tool, responsiveness focuses on the non-healthcare aspects of healthcare delivery, including the way in which patients are treated, the environment of that treatment, and the overall experience of the patient's contacts with the healthcare system.[4] Key indicators of responsiveness include attention, autonomy, amenities of care, choice, communication, confidentiality, and respect.[5] Table 4.2 applies these concepts in the context of Bosnia and Herzegovina. For a double function, the diagram also complements the recap of Bosnia's performance on the four hallmarks this chapter develops (see Table 4.1).

## Unveiling the Four Hallmarks

The four hallmarks of a good healthcare system are good laws, good funding, healthcare as a human right rather than a privilege, and good politics.[6] These factors are closely intertwined and separable only analytically rather than in a practical sense. Healthcare delivery is an onerous (but not an impossible) task because for a country to have a well-functioning healthcare system, all of these hallmarks must be present and converge.

The first hallmark of a good healthcare system is good laws. Many countries have a domestic legal system that includes its constitution (higher law) and the regional and international treaties relating to healthcare, notably the ICESCR, ratified by the country in question.

The second hallmark is good or adequate funding. Money is "the mother's milk of any healthcare system [. . .] and key to both access in healthcare and health outcomes."[7] Good funding, signified by the allocation of adequate revenue for healthcare services, is the lifeblood of a good healthcare system. The mark of the maturity of a state's healthcare system is the funding that, backed by the masses, the state's leaders are willing to devote to healthcare goods. A country can devote a sizable share of its gross domestic product (GDP) on healthcare, as the United States does,[8] and still get suboptimal healthcare results. However, adequate funding is an important starting point in the journey toward a good healthcare system.

How much a nation is willing to devote to healthcare, along with the level of material sacrifices it is ready to endure to get healthcare for the vast majority of its citizens—"opportunity cost," if we may—speaks to that nation's seriousness about improving healthcare. Few countries in the world have all the resources they need to meet their healthcare needs. Accordingly, achieving expanded healthcare requires the use of creative steps in funding, including efficient management of available resources and reducing waste.[9] Among other upsides, waste reduction makes it easier for health ministries to mount a successful argument before their ministries of finance for additional healthcare funding.[10]

Adequate funding is important because financial barriers impede access to healthcare services. Governments are obligated to protect individuals from impoverishment arising from illness, whether due to out-of-pocket payments or loss of income when a household member cannot work due to illness.[11] As then director-general of the WHO succinctly put it, "[n]o one in need of health care [. . .] should risk financial ruin as a result."[12] As people age, they become more susceptible to disease and disability; however, ill-health can afflict anyone at any age. Consequently, governments that are serious about making progress in reducing poverty must pay particular attention to providing quality access to good healthcare for most of their citizens.[13] In a nutshell, good healthcare financing requires "rais[ing] sufficient funds" for healthcare, minimizing "reliance on direct payments to finance services, and improv[ing] efficiency and equity."[14]

The third hallmark is healthcare as a human right rather than a privilege that the government may withdraw if it chooses. Human rights are guarantees of freedom, such as life, liberty, security, and subsistence to which people as human beings have rights.[15] Healthcare underpins many human rights, including the right to life; [16] thus, it may be viewed as the mother of socioeconomic human rights. However, just expanding healthcare does *not* automatically make it a human right; instead, the state in question must expressly make healthcare a human right within the law.[17] Thus, a country might make great strides toward universal healthcare and yet fail to afford its citizens the human right to healthcare. The United States exemplifies this scenario.[18] Expanded healthcare as a human right has several benefits, including an appeal to rights based solely on a person's humanity and a strategic push that can force governments to either hold the line on rights or increase those rights, rather than reduce them.[19]

Finally, the fourth hallmark of a good healthcare system is good politics. Healthcare is an "intrinsically political" phenomenon "built on principles of fairness and equity that require governments to allocate healthcare benefits according to need, and financial contributions according to ability to pay."[20] A transition to expanded healthcare is "primarily a political negotiation" between contending interest groups and stakeholders with divergent priorities, which may lead to "dysfunctional processes," if not handled well.[21] Accordingly, a government sends an important political message based on the healthcare funding it adopts.[22] Because "[i]n many countries the health care sector wields little political power or influence, decisions about the allocation of public funds[,]" "[e]xpenditure on health care has tended to be viewed simply as a drain on scarce resources, rather than as an investment in the nation's future."[23] Yet, policy decisions rooted in politics is part of the reason why "[c]ountries with similar levels of health expenditure achieve strikingly different health outcomes from their investment."[24]

"Health systems are one of the core areas of national responsibility" over which external actors can only provide a supporting role.[25] Therefore, as the World Health Organization advised, "any effective strategy for health financing needs to be home-grown."[26] This wisdom underlines the relationship between the two hallmarks of adequate funding and visionary leadership friendly to healthcare services in healthcare reforms. Going further, good politics has a distinctive characteristic that sets it apart from the other hallmarks in the sense that all of the other hallmarks—good laws, adequate funding, and healthcare as a human right—are susceptible to political influence. Put differently, at the risk of oversimplification, good politics may be viewed as a function of the previous three hallmarks, that is, politics designed to produce effective laws and adequate financing that increase the chances of making healthcare a human right rather than a privilege that a regime may withdraw when it chooses.

## ASSESSING BOSNIA'S PERFORMANCE ON THE FOUR HALLMARKS

The following discussion examines Bosnia's performance on the four hallmarks. Table 4.1 presents a diagram of the outcomes, with Table 4.2, cut from WHO assessment cloth, as a backup.

**Table 4.1**  Recap of Bosnia's performance on the four hallmarks

| Item no. | Hallmark | Key elements | Progress status | Bases for assessment |
|---|---|---|---|---|
| 1. | Good laws | Constitutionalization, ratification of multilateral treaty | Suboptimal | No role to state-level government |
| 2. | Good funding | Sufficient funding, minimizing reliance on direct payments to finance services, improve efficiency, and equity in healthcare financing | Suboptimal | Small size of GDP devoted to healthcare, low ratio of public spending, barriers posed by the poor state of the economy, and miscellaneous barriers somewhat related to funding |
| 3. | Health as human right | Entrenchment of features like expanded access, solidarity, and equity of a kind that makes healthcare a human right within the law | Suboptimal | Barriers from the three other hallmarks restrict movement of healthcare to human rights other than in a nominal sense |
| 4. | Good politics | Healthcare-friendly politics designed to produce effective laws and adequate financing that increase the chances of making healthcare a human right under the law | Suboptimal | Little success in diversifying funding of healthcare as a matter of politics. No consensus from politicians still steeped in ethnic security on any of the three possible approaches for diversification |

### Good Laws as Healthcare Reform in Bosnia

Chapter 2 noted an abiding yet abstract commitment to healthcare as a human right, evidenced in domestic and international laws, which dates back to socialist Yugoslavia. For Bosnia, good laws as healthcare signifies an area of comparative advantage that needs to be built upon with respect to genetic counseling, as elaborated in Chap. 7. For now, two points need to be kept in mind with regard to this hallmark. First, good laws as healthcare is not a one-time event, but rather an issue of constant improvement, not easily separated from the other hallmarks, particularly healthcare as a human right, and healthcare as good politics. Second, Bosnia does *not*

**Table 4.2** Health system statuses and performances of WHO members in 2000 (estimates for 1997), ranked by eight indicators: Juxtaposition of Bosnia with ten neighboring and non-neighboring countries

| Country | Health level (DALE)[a] | Health distribution | Responsiveness level | Responsiveness distribution | Fairness in financial contribution | Healthcare expenses per capita in US$ | Overall goal status[b] | Level of health performance | Ranking of health system |
|---|---|---|---|---|---|---|---|---|---|
| France | 3 | 12 | 16–17 | 3–38 | 26–29 | 4 | 6 | 4 | 1 |
| Italy | 6 | 14 | 22–23 | 3–38 | 45–47 | 11 | 11 | 3 | 2 |
| UK | 14 | 2 | 26–27 | 3–38 | 8–11 | 26 | 9 | 24 | 18 |
| USA | 24 | 32 | 1 | 3–38 | 54–55 | 1 | 15 | 72 | 37 |
| Slovenia | 34 | 23 | 37 | 53–57 | 82–83 | 29 | 29 | 62 | 38 |
| Croatia | 38 | 33 | 76–79 | 83 | 108–111 | 56 | 36 | 57 | 43 |
| Turkey | 73 | 109 | 93 | 66 | 49–50 | 82 | 96 | 33 | 70 |
| Macedonia[c] | 64 | 85 | 111 | 95 | 116–120 | 106 | 89 | 69 | 89 |
| **Bosnia** | **56** | **79** | **108–10** | **124** | **82–83** | **105** | **79** | **70** | **90** |
| Yugoslavia (Serbia and Montenegro)[d] | 46 | 90 | 115–117 | 116 | 158 | 113 | 95 | 47 | 106 |
| Myanmar (Burma) | 139 | 162 | 151–153 | 158 | 190 | 136 | 175 | 129 | 190 |
| Sierra Leone | 191 | 186 | 173 | 186 | 191 | 183 | 191 | 183 | 191 |

World Health Organization, *The World Health Report 2000: Health Systems: Improving Performance* (Geneva: World Health Organization, 2000), 152–55 (Annex, tbl. 1)

[a]DALE is the acronym for Disability-Adjusted Life Expectancy. It is "health equality in terms of child survival." Ibid., p. 144. Put differently, the term reports achievement on the average level of population health. Ibid., p. 146. It is "most easily understood as the expectation of life lived in equivalent full health." Ibid. The term is similar but not identical to Disability-Adjusted Life Year (DALY) used later in Chap. 7

[b]Regarding this information, the WHO explained that "[m]aximum attainable composite goal achievement was estimated using frontier production model

relating overall health system achievement to health expenditure and other non-health system determinants represented by educational attainment." World Health Organization, *The World Health Report 2000: Health Systems: Improving Performance* (Geneva: World Health Organization, 2000), 150

ᶜMacedonia became a member of the United Nations in April 1993. However, as a result of a dispute with Greece over the name Macedonia, the country was admitted under the provisional name of the former Yugoslav Republic of Macedonia, abbreviated as FYR Macedonia or FYROM. In June of 2018, Macedonia and Greece resolved the dispute with an agreement that the country should rename itself Republic of North Macedonia. This renaming came into effect in February 2019. See "North Macedonia," Cent. Intelligence, *The World Factbook*, https://www.cia.gov/library/publications/the-world-factbook/geos/mk.html

ᵈFollowing the death of Josip B. Tito in 1980, four republics, including BiH, separated from the state to form their own independent countries, leaving Serbia and Montenegro as the only two republics left of what used to be Yugoslavia. The two entities finally parted ways in June 2006 when, as a result of a referendum on independence in May, Montenegro voted to become a separate country. See Borga Brunner & David Johnson, "Timeline: Former Yugoslavia: From World War I to the Splintering of the Country," *Infoplease* (updated February 28, 2017), https://www.infoplease.com/history/world/timeline-the-former-yugoslavia

assign the state-level government a role in healthcare that complements the efforts at the entity and sub-entity levels.[27] This is an anomaly that calls for urgent rectification or remediation.

### Good Funding as Healthcare Reform in Bosnia

BiH ranks even worse on this benchmark than it does on good laws. Numerous interlinked factors related to funding which impede healthcare in Bosnia and Herzegovina include the following: an inadequate share of the gross domestic product devoted to healthcare; a low ratio of public spending on healthcare, relative to its neighbors, inconsistent with the concept of expanded healthcare; and the poor state of the BiH economy. A fourth set of factors, a number of them bureaucratic, completes this list of barriers in funding. No thanks to these funding issues, "[a]t the current levels of treatment, the lives of persons in need of medical treatment for chronic diseases or conditions, even if these would not ordinarily be considered life threatening conditions outside BiH, may be jeopardized if they are forced to seek treatment in BiH."[28] The net effect is that, despite the promise of a compulsory health insurance program funded by the state, many residents live with nominal health coverage and forego expensive private medical services they are not able to pay for.[29]

#### Small Size of the GDP Devoted to Healthcare

Bosnia spends less than 10% of its GDP on healthcare, a threshold that many healthcare experts consider ideal.[30] WHO figures for 2014 (the most recent year for which information is available) show that BiH devoted only 9.6% of its GDP to healthcare.[31] Although seemingly respectable, the figure is below the numbers for European countries like Austria, Belgium, Denmark, France, Germany, the Netherlands, Sweden, and Switzerland. Each of these countries allocates more than 10% of its GDP to healthcare. [32] With many lingering problems from the war that need to be addressed, BiH's single-digit allocations to healthcare are insufficient.

#### Low Ratio of Public Spending on Healthcare

Indicative of the low outlay for healthcare in BiH is the low *public* healthcare spending per capita versus the relatively high *private* healthcare spending per capita. Based on WHO data, in 2014, BiH's public spending per capita on healthcare was US$464.[33] In 2015, 71% of total healthcare spending (amounting to 1.895 million Bosnian Convertible Mark (KM),[34] out of 2.669 billion KM) was public, while 29% (amounting to 774 million KM) was private.[35] This is probably due to the country's low GDP.[36] Regardless, the ratio of public spending to private spending is rather low, compared to European countries like Denmark, Germany, the Netherlands, and Norway, whose expenditures are about ten to twenty times higher per capita.[37] The increased private expenditure was particularly noticeable in areas like dentistry, diagnostics, over-the-counter drugs, as well as therapeutic and specialist services.[38] Moreover, the gap in expenditure in favor of the private sector results in investment in equipment, new technologies, and services, which often draws people to private or overseas healthcare institutions, instead of public ones.[39]

Note that public funding here does *not* mean budget funds. Instead, it comprises mostly compulsory health insurance funds from workers' contributions, analyzed in Chap. 3 with budget funds covering about 9% of public expenditure and 6% of total expenditures.[40] These funds are mainly used for capital investments, public health, and preventive initiatives.[41] Under the current system, employers and their employees bear the burden of financing health insurance. They are the only sections of the populace contributing financially to the public healthcare system. Unlike other categories (such as the unemployed, pensioners, students, and farmers), employers and employees pay more than their share in the population of insured people.[42] Additionally, BiH has a highly informal economy, estimated at between 25% and 57% of the GDP, that generates no public revenues for the healthcare sector.[43] In short, under BiH's current system of healthcare financing, the surplus from employed persons' contributions covers the deficit of revenues generated by all other insured categories, even though the employed group makes up only slightly over one-third of the insured population.[44] For example, as shown with RS data on Table 3.2 in Chap. 3, from 2014 to 2018, employees comprised slightly over 35% of the total number of insured categories but contributed almost 84% of the total public revenue.

Juxtaposed with other countries', Bosnia's budget share for financing total healthcare expenditure ranks among the lowest.[45] For example, compared to twenty-nine other European countries, Bosnia ranked seventeenth in 2014.[46] This was part of a longitudinal survey on public health sector expenditure from 1995 to 2014 where, in 2014, Bosnia averaged 71.2%,[47] a figure below the European average of 76.2%.[48] The Netherlands placed first with 87% and Albania last with 49.9%.[49] Copays that insured persons must pay when they see a doctor, innocuously passed off as "participatory fees," threaten financial ruin for a broad section of the population.[50] "[O]ut-of-pocket payments for healthcare are those contributions [that] the poorest households and people usually cannot afford," which is often why these individuals delay or forego treatment.[51] In 2014, these payments accounted for approximately 97% of private contributions for healthcare services.[52] The high number imposes a serious burden on families living near or below the poverty line.[53] It also means that about half a million people delay purchasing medicines they need or seeking healthcare services, inconsistent with preventive medicine.[54] This is a heavy burden for this group of people, which impedes their ability to escape poverty.[55]

*Impediment Posed by the Poor State of the Bosnian Economy*
Bosnia's dire economic condition complicates the inadequate public funding of healthcare in the country. In 2017, the Office of High Representative, which exercises oversight over the country to ensure it does not relapse into war, in economic terms, assessed "a[n] [economic] decline across several areas," in the country, compared to its neighbors.[56] That year, BiH had a GDP of US$18.08 billion,[57] with a per capita income of US$5827.[58] While on the surface these numbers seem modest for a small country still reeling from the effects of a bloody ethnic war, the figures conceal suboptimal score on several key economic indicators, such as foreign direct investment (DFI),[59] the index of economic freedom,[60] ease of doing business,[61] human development,[62] global competitiveness,[63] and credit rating.[64] Additionally, BiH has an inefficient public sector,[65] a high unemployment rate,[66] high poverty rate,[67] large-scale emigration from the country,[68] a large informal sector,[69] large-scale corruption,[70] and suffers from consumption of goods and services at a higher rate than it produces.[71] BiH also borrows extensively domestically and internationally, and it relies heavily on foreign aid.[72] The bottom line is that, although the World Bank ranks BiH as an "upper middle income" country, compared to many of its neighbors in Europe, in many respects Bosnia is still a poor country,[73] with negative ramifications for healthcare and preventive medicine.

*Miscellaneous Impediments Somewhat Related to Funding*
Miscellaneous problems more or less tied to inadequate funding which impede healthcare services in Bosnia include the following: difficulties insured persons face when they try to take their coverage with them when

they move to a residence outside of their registered area;[74] absence of any obligation by Cantonal Funds to transfer resources or data to FBiH Health Insurance Fund;[75] failure of an affected contributing agency (i.e., company or institution) to pay its contribution(s) into an affected healthcare fund;[76] absence of inter-entity or inter-cantonal cooperation;[77] and "undermin[ing] the effective operation of the principle of a common pool of resources and of commonly-shared risks" created by the existence of thirteen disparate healthcare systems' health funds (counting the two entities alone, without the Brčko administrative district).[78] Other impediments somewhat related to funding are the following: lack of cooperation among the different healthcare jurisdictions on issues bearing on healthcare delivery;[79] a primary healthcare system designed to cover 70–80% of all medical cases that, in actuality, processed only 10–20% of the projected volume;[80] transportation problems due to a rugged topography;[81] and an emergency system that does not function well.[82]

Similarly, Bosnia "does not have sufficient pharmaceutical manufacturing to cover its entire needs," leading to dependence on importing drugs to satisfy those unmet needs.[83] Neither the country's two entities nor the self-governing unit comes close to the ranges in drug quantity, 250–350, that the WHO recommends as ideal on the Essential Drug List (EDL).[84] Instead, of the recommended range, FBiH maintained only a list of about 160 drugs and RS boasted a PL of 105, while Brčko District had neither an EDL nor PL.[85]

### Human Right as Healthcare Reform in Bosnia

Healthcare as a human right is antithetical to the idea of healthcare as a privilege—a revocable gift from the government. As the discussion in Chap. 2 pointed out, Bosnia integrated former Yugoslavia's socialist approach of treating healthcare as a human right. The only question is to what extent BiH citizens may enjoy that right. The European Union identifies several values in healthcare delivery—universality, access to high-quality healthcare, solidarity, and equity.[86] In gauging healthcare as human rights, these values can serve handily as proxies. In 2015, Bosnia scored little over 78% on the Healthcare Access and Quality Index (HAQ).[87] The HAQ Index is measured on a scale from 0 (worst) to 100, based on death rates from thirty-two causes of death that could have been avoided by timely and effective medical treatment.[88] While on its face 78% on HAQ appears respectable, here, as in several other matters of human development, Bosnia ranks below its neighbors.[89] Going further, in 2017, Bosnia compiled 1.16 out of a possible 5.4 points on the Human Rights Score.[90] Based on the ethic of human rights, as one analyst poignantly put it, "[t]he goal of a healthcare system [should be] to enhance the health of the population in the most effective manner possible in light of a society's available resources and competing needs."[91] The same ethic presages the proper role for politics in healthcare reforms, elaborated next below.

### Good Politics as Healthcare Reform in Bosnia

There is little indication that Bosnian political leaders are treating healthcare as a high priority on their policy agenda. Over the years, political actors have pushed for healthcare financing reform.[92] This reform entails shifting away from excessive dependence on workers' contributions due to the following factors: a low share of employed persons in an aging population, high unemployment rates, increased demand for healthcare services, a low-average salary, and a deficit in healthcare funding caused by rising healthcare costs.[93] With respect to the deficit, in 2015, the Federation of Bosnia and Herzegovina and its ten cantons faced a problem of illiquidity that amounted to more than 120 million KM (about €60 million) in total unpaid claims of funds,[94] while its co-entity, Republika Srpska, had a loss of more than 20 million KM (about €10 million).[95]

These factors leave the healthcare system vulnerable to economic recessions, which affect the availability of funds and create financial insecurity.[96] The same factors also call for diversifying sources of healthcare funding by integrating non-contribution revenues into a system that relies on contributions based largely on wages.[97] Martić and Đukić proposed three possible roads to achieve diversification,[98] that the following discussion reviews, together with the role of good politics in each option. In Bosnia, diversification is already underway, but the process has yet to yield tangible and observable results.[99]

### Diversification Through Minor Adjustments (i.e., Reallocating and Earmarking) of the Current System

The first way to achieve diversification is "ensuring alternative revenue sources [while] maintaining the same level of contribution rates."[100] The imagery this model brings to mind is mending the system as we know it, rather than ending it. Under this arrangement, alternative revenues are provided by reallocating budget funds to increase the health insurance funds or by introducing additional earmarked revenue sources, such as "new excise duties on tobacco, alcohol, fuel, harmful soft drinks, and luxur[y] products."[101] As Martić and Đukić explain, taxes earmarked for harmful products help reduce their use and provide additional funds for financing treatment costs incurred because of consuming such products.[102] Under this approach, good politics will serve the role of prioritizing funds for healthcare and efficiently utilizing available revenue. It is the lowest hanging fruit among the three options that has, however, yet to emerge.

*Diversification Through Tax Restructuring of the Current System*
The second way to achieve diversification is through tax restructuring. Under this model, alternative sources of revenue is provided for healthcare by reducing the required health insurance contributions employees must currently pay from their salaries.[103] This option may include an increase in excise taxes on tobacco and alcohol.[104] It may also include additional alternative revenues, such as those generated by increasing indirect taxes, like the value-added tax (VAT) and property taxes.[105] Like the first method, this second way of achieving diversification is predicated on good politics that prioritizes healthcare funding, reduces wastefulness, and combats corruption. But, unlike the first option, it is also a diversification route a notch higher in progressiveness that calls for more discipline, creative bipartisanship, and political will than Bosnian politicians, steeped in "ethnic security" twenty-five years after the war,[106] can muster.

*Diversification Through Complete Restructuring of the Current System*
The third possible means of diversification of healthcare funding on the list of proposals by Martić and Đukić is diversification through complete restructure of the current healthcare financing model by transitioning to financing healthcare with budget revenues.[107] Under this approach, all citizens would be entitled to access state-sponsored healthcare without any prerequisites,[108] with two caveats: it would *not* preclude people from obtaining private insurance if they need extra coverage, and it would *not* preclude burdensome copays.[109] Even though this option does not increase individuals' health insurance contributions, it does not forbid increasing direct or indirect taxes.[110] In proposing these ways of diversifying revenue sources, Martić and Đukić noted that their calculations did not explain how to collect funds and contract with service providers or what role the private sector should play;[111] the authors advised supporting reforms for each of these.[112] This observation calls for political involvement. If Bosnian

politicians succeed in accomplishing reforms, they will curtail "the burden on labor needs" that, among other pledges, they promised to implement in the Reform Agenda for Bosnia and Herzegovina 2015–2018.[113]

Compared to the first two approach, this last category signifies a clean break from the past, and ending the current system as we know it, rather than mending it. Unlike the first two, this approach assigns politics the highest role in healthcare decision-making, and, because, more than the other competing approaches, it promotes the principles of universality, equality, and solidarity in the distribution of healthcare goods, this model draws Bosnia closest to the reality of healthcare as a human right.[114] But this model demands more political capital that, from the look of things, just doesn't exist in Bosnia and may not be for some time to come, given the political divisiveness embedded in resort to the comfort of ethnic security that marks Bosnian politics twenty-five years after the war.[115]

This chapter sets forth a guide for healthcare reforms in Bosnia that is built on four hallmarks, including a ranking of Bosnia's performance on those benchmarks. Without exception, the performance was mixed on all fronts—effective laws, adequate funding with solid plans for diversification of healthcare funding, traction on the road to healthcare as human right, and politics friendly and conducive to quality and affordable healthcare. This result was disappointing in all aspects (see Table 4.1). Take good politics which, as indicated earlier, can have a spillover effect over the other hallmarks.[116] Testament to the "dysfunctional processes," inconsonant with healthcare administration,[117] that still occur in Bosnia twenty-five years after the war is the fact that a politician's suggestion for reform recently triggered disagreeable "political reactions" in the Federation of Bosnia and Herzegovina,[118] the larger of the country's two entities.

There is no perfect or error-safe system for assessing the status and performance of healthcare systems. In its 2000 report, WHO portrayed the wealth of information that it presented as "innovative" materials that "can be refined and improved," and expressed the hope that "careful scrutiny and use of the results will lead to progressively better measurements" in the future.[119] For the measures of responsiveness and equity in financial contributions wherein it used a range, rather than exact figures, WHO explained that "[a]ll the main results are reported with uncertainty intervals in order to communicate to the user the plausible range of estimates for each country on each measure."[120] Worse still, WHO used estimates for 1997, three years behind the publication of its report and some of the healthcare systems like Serbia and Montenegro (the two remaining republics in Yugoslavia after four left) became nonexistent years after the report. Little wonder perhaps that after its ranking in 2000, the global health czar stopped producing these rankings, citing "the complexity of the task."[121] The same sense of humility informs the hallmarks this chapter develops. The same sense of humility explains the characterization and (re)presentation of the hallmarks in the foregoing analysis as a guide. The conversation in this chapter was designed as a prelude to the analysis in the next part of the book on preventive medicine, made up of three complementary chapters, Chaps. 5, 6, and 7. The searchlight turns next to that theme, beginning with Chap. 5, which defines genetic counseling.

## NOTES

1. See Marc J. Roberts et al., *Getting Health Reform Right: A Guide to Improving Performance and Equity* (New York: Oxford Univ. Press, 2008). The book also discussed other methods for measuring the performance of healthcare systems, including models based on economics. Different characteristics (means) and frameworks abound for comparing healthcare systems. There are about seven of the characteristics altogether. These include the following: (i) the organization, financing, and control of a healthcare system; (ii) physician characteristics and provider arrangements for primary care and prevention; (iii) hospitals and long-term care arrangements; and (iv) the degree to which healthcare is integrated and coordinated between various sectors and levels of service. Others are: (v) economic characteristics, personnel resources, utilization rates, and population health status measures; (vi) specific problems, such as assessments of citizen satisfaction; and (vii) strategies for reform. The first breaks down into whether a government owns the means of producing healthcare, whether it acts as the purchaser of healthcare services, or whether it takes the role of overseer (e.g., setting mandates for health coverage and regulating the terms) of what is largely a private system. The categories are not mutually exclusive, given that a government may assume more than one role in a particular system. For example, within the spectrum of the US market-based system, the Veteran Administration operates its own healthcare subsystem. Also "owning" the means of producing healthcare does not mean perfect ownership of a healthcare system. For example, in Sweden where the government takes it upon itself to provide healthcare, only about 85%, not 100% of healthcare services, is publicly funded. See Mary Ko Zimmerman, Comparative Health-Care Systems," *Encyclopedia of Sociology* (Updated Jan. 25, 2020), https://

60 P. C. AKA

www.encyclopedia.com/social-sciences/encyclopedias-almanacs-alma-
nacs-transcripts-and-maps/comparative-health-care-systems
2. See, for example, Philip C. Aka et al., "Ghana's National Health Insurance
Scheme (NHIS) and the Evolution of a Human Right to Healthcare in
Africa," *Chicago-Kent J. Int'l & Comp. Law*, 17(2) (2017), 1–65; José
M. Zuniga et al., eds., *Advancing the Human Right to Health* (New York:
Oxford University Press, 2013) (among other achievements, this edited
volume sought to provide an account of the parameters of the right to
health, strategies on ways to achieve this right, and discussion as to why
realization of the right is so essential in the twenty-first century).
3. See generally World Health Organization, *The World Health Report 2000:
Health Systems: Improving Performance* (Geneva: World Health
Organization, 2000).
4. See, for example, Bereket Yakob & Busisiwe Purity Ncama, "Measuring
Health System Responsiveness at Facility Level in Ethiopia: Performance,
Correlates[,] and Implications," 17 *BMC Health Service Research* (2017),
263, doi: https://doi.org/10.1186/s12913-017-2224-1.
5. Ibid.
6. Reference has been made earlier in this work to the inherent normative
tone of comparative healthcare studies. See Chap. 1, note 35, and accompanying text. Therefore, "good" is proxy for *optimalness* or *optimality,* a
heuristic standard in economic theory believed to be reached when
resources may not be "reallocated to make one individual better off without making at least one individual worse off." Jim Chappelow, "Pareto
Efficiency," *Investopedia* (updated Sept. 25, 2019), https://www.
investopedia.com/terms/p/pareto-efficiency.asp
7. Aka et al., note 2, pp. 1, 23.
8. Matej Mikulic, "Health Expenditure as a Percentage of Gross Domestic
Product in Selected Countries in 2017," *Statista* (last edited Aug. 9,
2019), https://www.statista.com/statistics/268826/health-expendi-
ture-as-gdp-percentage-in-oecd-countries/ (showing that the United
States expended 17.2% of its GDP in 2017 on healthcare). See also Lita
Epstein, "6 Reasons Healthcare Is So Expensive in the U.S.," *Investopedia*
(updated July 30, 2019), https://www.investopedia.com/articles/per-
sonal-finance/080615/6-reasons-healthcare-so-expensive-us.
asp,archived at https://perma.cc/YD8V-6TPN ("If the $3 trillion
U.S. healthcare sector were ranked as a country, it would be the world's
fifth largest economy[.]").
9. See "Executive Summary: Why Universal Coverage?" *in* World Health
Organization, *The World Health Report: Health Systems Financing: The
Path to Universal Coverage* (Geneva: 2010), ix–xxii.
10. Ibid., p. xi

11. World Health Organization, "What is Universal Coverage?" http://www.who.int/health_financing/universal_coverage_definition/en/
12. Margaret Chan, "Message from the Director-General," *in* World Health Organization, *The World Health Report: Health Systems Financing: The Path to Universal Coverage* (Geneva: 2010), vii.
13. See, for example, David H. Peters et al., "Poverty and Access to Health Care in Developing Countries," 1136 *Ann. N.Y. Acad. Sci.* (2008), 161–71, doi: https://doi.org/10.1196/annals.1425.011.
14. Chan, note 12.
15. See, for example, Jack Donnelly, *Universal Human Rights in Theory and Practice* (Ithaca, NY: Cornell Univ. Press, 3d. ed. 2013), 7–23 (analyzing the concept of human rights).
16. See generally World Health Organization, *Health in All Policies: Helsinki Statement Framework for Country Action* (Geneva: World Health Organization, 2014).
17. See generally Aka et al., note 2; Philip C. Aka, "Analyzing U.S. Commitment to Socioeconomic Human Rights," *Akron Law Rev.*, 39 (2006), 417–63.
18. See, for example, Hector Florimon, "Why the US Spends More on Health Care Than Other Countries, But Doesn't Fare Better: Study," *ABC News* (Sept. 12, 2019, 7.45 PM), https://abcnews.go.com/Health/us-spends-health-care-countries-fare-study/story?id=53710650 (putting some of the blame on prescription drugs). According to this analyst, "[i]n the U.S. people spend, per person, nearly double the on pharmaceutical drugs – $1443 – compared to the average of other countries, $749." Ibid.
19. Aka et al., note 2, pp. 27–35.
20. David Heymann & Robert Yates, "Embracing the Politics of Universal Health Coverage," *Chatham House* (June 25, 2014), https://www.chathamhouse.org/expert/comment/embracing-politics-universal-health-coverage, archived at https://perma.cc/65KF-K5LV
21. Chan, note 12, pp. vi, vii.
22. Marko Martić & Ognjen Đukić, Friedrich Ebert Stiftung Sarajevo, "Health Care System in BiH: Financing Challenges and Reform Options? (Oct. 2017), 22–23. See also ibid., p. 27 (stating, citing Croatia and Slovenia, that "the legacy of the former [Yugoslavia] has a strong influence on the current models.").
23. World Health Organization, *World Health Report 1995: Bridging the Gaps* (Geneva: World Health Organization, 1995), 91.
24. Chan, note 12, p. vii.
25. Nick Fahy, "Commentary on International Health System Performance Information," *in* Irene Papanicolas & Peter C. Smith, eds., *Health System*

*Performance Comparison: An Agenda for Policy, Information and Research* (England: Open Univ. Press, 2013), 313–14.

26. Chan, note 12, p. vii.

27. See Chap. 1 (Introduction) and Chap. 7 ("Last Word on Reforms").

28. United Nations High Commissioner for Refugees' Office of the Chief of Mission in Bosnia, *Health Care in Bosnia and Herzegovina in the Context of the Return of Refugees and Displaced Persons* (Sarajevo: July 2001) [hereinafter *Health Care in BiH*], p. i.

29. Ibid., pp. i, 1.

30. See, for example, William D. Savedoff, "What Should a Country Spend on Health Care," *Health Affairs*, 26(4) (2007), 962–70, https://www.healthaffairs.org/doi/pdf/10.1377/hlthaff.26.4.962 (noting the WHO's suggestion of 5%, but going beyond the recommendation to consider four approaches—peer, political economy, production function, and budget—after which Savedoff settled on the budget approach as the most feasible and readily quantifiable). See also the Abuja Declaration of 2001: World Health Organization, "The Abuja Declaration: Ten Years On" (2011), https://www.who.int/healthsystems/publications/abuja_declaration/en/ (suggesting a target of 15% of the annual budget of the African countries which adopted the declaration in the Nigerian capital, which target only one country reached ten years later in 2011).

31. World Bank, "Health Expenditure Total (% of GDP)," https://data.worldbank.org/indicator/SH.XPD.TOTL.ZS

32. Martić and Đukić, note 22, p. 10. The precise numbers for France and Germany, respectively, are 11.5% and Germany 11.3% and the United States, not as model for BiH but only as nominal benchmark at 17.1% of GDP. Ibid.

33. Ibid., p. 11 (citing WHO data for 2014).

34. Ibid., p. 9. The KM is the local abbreviation of the Bosnian and Herzegovina Convertible Mark (BAM), the Bosnian currency. *BAM - Bosnian Convertible Mark*, xe, https://www.xe.com/currency/bam-bosnian-convertible-mark, *archived at* https://perma.cc/8BLB-6N9Z. As of May 2020, 1 KM exchanges for 55 cents US currency.

35. Martić and Đukić, note 22, pp. 9, 17. Private sources include various forms of participation, direct payments for drugs and other therapeutic aids, as well as informal (i.e., unlawful) payments for medical services. Ibid., p. 17, n. 13. More than 50% of the private expenditure in healthcare in BiH goes into medical treatment services, followed by medical supplies for outpatient care services, financed mainly from private resources, and ancillary healthcare services, and so forth. Ibid., p.10. Medicines and therapeutic aids formed the biggest share of household (suggesting that the approved list of medication does not have them). Of

the amount spent on out-of-hospital dental protections in BiH, 65% was funded from private sources, suggesting that many citizens use the services of private dental practitioners. Ibid.

36. Ibid., p. 9.
37. Ibid. Compared to its neighbors, in 2014, BiH's *private* healthcare spending was 2.76% of GDP—over and above 1.4% of GDP for Croatia, 2.6% of GDP for Slovenia, and the EU average of 2.2%. Ibid., p. 11. Similarly, in 2014, the share of private expenditure in total health expenditure in BiH was 28%, double the EU average of 14%. Martić and Đukić, note 22, p. 1.
38. Ibid., p. 13.
39. Ibid.
40. Ibid., p. 19. See also ibid., p. 18, tbl. 5, indicating a share of total expenditure of 0.02% for budget of BiH institutions, 3.5% for budget of entities, and 2.9% for budgets of cantons.
41. Martić and Đukić, note 22, p. 19.
42. Ibid., 19 & tbl. 6.
43. Ibid., p. 19.
44. Ibid.
45. Ibid.
46. Ibid., p. 17.
47. Ibid., p. 17 (chart 10).
48. Ibid., p. 17.
49. Ibid.
50. Ibid., pp. 21–22 (discussing the negative impacts of out-of-pocket payments on the poor).
51. Ibid., p. 21.
52. Ibid., p. 21, n.20. Items like voluntary health insurance completed the remainder. Ibid., p. 21.
53. Ibid., p. 21.
54. Ibid., p. 22.
55. Ibid.
56. Office of the High Representative, Fifty-First Report of the High Representative for Implementation of the Peace Agreement on Bosnia and Herzegovina to the Secretary-General of the United Nations (May 17, 2017) [hereinafter Fifty-First Report on BiH] (Part VIII. Economy), http://www.ohr.int/?p=97409. *The General Framework Agreement for Peace in Bosnia and Herzegovina*, Yugoslavia—Bosn. & Herz.—Croatia, December 14, 1995 [hereinafter *Dayton Peace Agreement*] (more popularly known as the Dayton Peace Agreement), which ended the Bosnian conflict of 1992 to 1995, gave the High Representative the power to implement the civilian side of that agreement. See Dayton Peace

Agreement, note 56, Art. VIII, Annex 10 (agreement on civilian implementation).

57. "Bosnia and Herzegovina GDP," *Trading Econ.*, https://tradingeconomics.com/bosnia-and-herzegovina/gdp, *archived at* https://perma.cc/Y6DD-H3WQ

58. "Bosnia and Herzegovina GDP Per Capita," *Trading Econ.*, https://tradingeconomics.com/bosnia-and-herzegovina/gdp-per-capita, archived at https://perma.cc/Q8CF-PY45

59. Fifty-First Report on BiH, note 56 (Part VIII. Economy) (recounting that, in 2016, BiH ranked fourth in foreign direct investment inflows in Southeastern Europe on the UN Conference on Trade and Development's World Investment Report). See also Council of Europe, Parliamentary Assembly, *The Honoring of Obligations and Commitments by Bosnia and Herzegovina* (Doc. No. 14465) (January 8, 2018), 7 ¶ 10 [hereinafter *Honoring Obligations by BiH*]. (January 8, 2018) (stating that DFI decreased from 2.69% of GDP in 2014 to 1.67% in 2015).

60. Fifty-First Report of the High Representative, note 56 (Part VIII. Economy) (indicating that, in 2016, BiH ranked 109th out of 178 countries in the world, 39th out of 43 in Europe on the Heritage Foundations Index of Economic Freedom for 2016, and 91st out of 159 economies on the Economic Freedom of the World Annual Report for 2016).

61. Fifty-First Report of the High Representative, note 56 (Part VIII. Economy) (stating that BiH ranked 81st out of 190 countries on the World Bank's Doing Business Report in 2017, "the worst of all Balkan countries.")

62. The country ranked 75th out of 189 countries in the 2018 UNDP's Human Development Report. See *United Nations Dev. Program, Inequalities in Human Development in the twenty-first Century: Bosnia and Herzegovina* (Mar. 30, 2020), 2, http://hdr.undp.org/sites/all/themes/hdr_theme/country-notes/BIH.pdf. This was a slight improvement from 2015, when it ranked 85th out of 188 countries. Fifty-First Report on BiH, note 56 (Part VIII. Economy).

63. Fifty-First Report of the High Representative, note 56 (Part VIII. Economy) (observing that BiH ranked 107th out of 138 economies, the lowest in the Balkan region, on the World Economic Forum's Global Competitiveness Report for 2016–2017).

64. Ibid. (observing that, in 2017, BiH ranked "B with stable outlook" on the Standard and Poor's Rating Services, based on factors like fiscal performance, robust indirect tax revenues, and debt burden,).

65. *Honoring Obligations by BiH*, note 59, p. 7 ¶ 9. See also Ellen Goldstein et al., "Three Reasons Why the Economy of Bosnia and Herzegovina Is

Off Balance," *Brookings: Future Development* (Nov. 5, 2015), https://www.brookings.edu/blog/future-development/2015/11/05/three-reasons-why-the-economy-of-bosnia-and-herzegovina-is-off-balance/ (counting a large public sector that constricts creation of private wealth among three major, mutually reinforcing, imbalances that the country needs to correct).

66. See *Honoring Obligations by BiH*, note 59, p. 7 ¶ 9 (putting the number at 27.7% of the working population). This is especially problematic among the youth. *Id.* (indicating that about 60% or six out of every ten youths are unemployed). Such a phenomenon has resulted in political corruption associated with job search. The Council of Europe's report cites a case in point involving the Secretary-General of the Party of Democratic Action (SDA), who was arrested in February 2017 for selling jobs in public companies. Ibid., p. 7 ¶ 9 & n.5. According to the report, a job as an electrician for Elektoprivredra, the public electricity company, sold for €8000. Ibid., p. 7 n.5.

67. See *Honoring Obligations by BiH*, note 59, p. 7, ¶ 9, n.5. (putting the share of the population living below the poverty line as 48%). A fallout from this is that many Bosnians depend on remittances from abroad as a significant source of income. Ibid., p. 7, ¶ 10 (US$1347.93 million in 2015, quoting the World Bank). See also Goldstein et al., note 65 (noting that about 20% of the country's GDP came from other financial inflows like foreign aid and remittances).

68. See *Honoring Obligations by BiH*, note 59, p. 7 ¶ 9 (noting one reason people are leaving is because of the scarcity of employment); *see also* Fifty-First Report on BiH, note 56 (Part VIII. Economy) (stating that on the World Economic Forum's Global Competitiveness Report for 2016–2017, BiH ranked 134th out of 138 countries regarding the capacity to retain talent).

69. BiH's informal economy is estimated at 25–37% of the country's GDP. Andreja Živković, *Balkan Monitoring Pub. Finances, Analysis on Tax Justice: Bosnia and Herzegovina* (September 2017), 6. This article defines "informal" broadly to include indicators such as when taxable income for social security is paid at the minimum wage level, although the actual salary was higher; taxable income for social security is reported as lower than the actual income paid; actual payment is higher than that written in the contract; no health insurance is provided on the main job; no social security payment is given on the main job; and when there is no written contract for the main job. Ibid., p. 10.

70. Fifty-First Report on BiH, note 56 (Part VIII. Economy) (observing that in Transparency International's Corruption Perceptions Index for 2015, BiH ranked 83rd out of 176 countries).

71. *Honoring Obligations by BiH*, note 59, p. 7 ¶ 9 & n.4 (noting that, in 2014, imports represented 56.9% of BiH's GDP, while exports accounted for only 33.9%); Goldstein et al., note 65 ("Exports are worth only 30 percent of GDP, one of the lowest in Europe [. . . .] If BiH exported as much as it did during Yugoslav times, its exports would be three times as high.").
72. *Honoring Obligations by BiH*, note 59, p. 7, ¶ 10. According to this report, BiH maintains foreign currency reserves large enough to cover imports for six months. Ibid., p. 7, ¶ 11.
73. Based on the World Bank's figure of $4,616 USD GDP per capita that the Council of Europe used, BiH has a 28% purchasing power per capita, which is lower than Albania's 30%, Serbia's 36%, Croatia's 58%, and Slovenia's 83%. *Honoring Obligations by BiH*, note 59, 7 & n.3.
74. *Health Care in BiH*, note 28, pp. 6–7, 23.
75. Ibid., p. i, 7–9.
76. Ibid.
77. Ibid.
78. Ibid., p. 23.
79. Ibid., pp. i, 1.
80. Ibid., p. i, 1, 25 (referring to FBiH, one of the two entities that make up the country).
81. Ibid., p. i. See also ibid., pp. 27–8 (commenting on the physical-environmental conditions impeding healthcare delivery in BiH).
82. Ibid., p. 51 (pointing out that the country has "less than [one] vehicle per 100,000 inhabitants," with the result that in places where an ambulance is available, "it can take up to 3 hours for an emergency vehicle to arrive on-site following a call.").
83. Jennifer Cain et al., eds., *Health Care Systems in Transition: Bosnia and Herzegovina* (Copenhagen: European Observatory on Health Care Systems, 2002), 76.
84. *Health Care in BiH*, note 28, p. 28. The EDL is the quantity of drugs that the WHO recommends should be available free of charge in all countries as a basic standard of treatment. Ibid. From this standard, BiH has distilled a Positive List (PL), that is, a list of drugs which must be on hand in state pharmacies or related healthcare outfits available to patients free of charge or subject to a small copay euphemistically known in BiH as "participation fee." Ibid.
85. Ibid. (data as of 2000).
86. Martić and Đukić, note 22, p. 5. In the context the European Union used them, *universality* means that no one is denied access to healthcare; *access* is present when healthcare is within reach or affordable, free of non-

burdensome barriers; *solidarity* denotes the need to ensure access to healthcare for all; and *equity* stands for equal access based on need, without discrimination based on gender, age, social status, or ability to pay. See ibid.

87. "Bosnia and Herzegovina: Healthcare Access and Quality Index, 1990 to 2015," *Our World in Data*, https://ourworldindata.org/grapher/healthcare-access-and-quality-index?tab=chart&country=BIH (the exact number was 78.2%).

88. Ibid.

89. In the Human Development Report for 2019 (based on data for 2018), BiH scored approximately 0.77 in the "high human development" category, compared, for example, to Turkey (approximately 0.81), Montenegro (approximately 0.82), Croatia (approximately 0.84), and Slovenia (little over 0.90) in the "very high human development" category. See *Human Development Report 2019: Beyond Income, Beyond Averages, Beyond Today: Inequalities in Human Development in the twenty-first Century* (New York: United Nations Dev. Program, 2019).

90. "Bosnia and Herzegovina: Human Rights Score, 1992 to 2017," *Our Word in Data*, https://ourworldindata.org/grapher/human-rights-scores?tab=chart&time=1992.2017&country=BIH. Similarly, in 2014, Bosnia earned an uninspiring 6.1 out of a possible 10 points in the Human Rights Violations Index. The index is a composite metric based on multiple variables, including press freedom, political freedoms religious freedom, human trafficking, and torture, among other variables. "Bosnia and Herzegovina: Human Rights Violations, 2006 to 2014," *Our World in Data*, https://ourworldindata.org/grapher/human-rights-violations?tab=chart&country=BIH. Concededly, these two measures belong mostly in the realm of political-civil rights, and bear only a tangential connection to the socioeconomic human right to healthcare at the heart of this book.

91. I. Gregory Pawlson et al., "Healthcare Systems," *Encyclopedia of Bioethics* (Updated December 4, 2019), https://www.encyclopedia.com/science/encyclopedias-almanacs-transcripts-and-maps/healthcare-systems

92. See Martić and Đukić, note 22, pp. 25–6 (discussing current initiatives for reforming health financing schemes).

93. Ibid., pp. 5, 26.

94. Ibid., p. 17.

95. Ibid., p. 15.

96. Ibid., p. 19.

97. Ibid., pp. 23, 24, 28. Diversification serves the same purpose of inoculation against excessive exposure to risk as it does in investment. It is "a risk

management strategy that mixes a wide variety of investments within a portfolio. The rationale behind this technique is that a portfolio constructed of different kinds of assets will, on average, yield higher long-term returns and lower the risk of any individual holding or security." Troy Segal, "Diversification," *Investopedia*, https://www.investopedia.com/terms/d/diversification.asp, *archived at* https://perma.cc/7XED-DSVY. "Diversification strives to smooth out unsystematic risk events in a portfolio, [such that] the positive performance of some investments neutralizes the negative performance of others." Ibid.

98. Martić and Đukić, note 22, pp. 28–9.
99. Ibid., p. 28.
100. Ibid.
101. Ibid.
102. Ibid.
103. Ibid.
104. Ibid.
105. Ibid.
106. See, for example, Vesna Bojicic-Dzelilovic, "The Politics, Practice[,] and Paradox of 'Ethnic Security' in Bosnia-Herzegovina," *Stability: Int'l J. Security & Dev.*, 4(1) (2015), Art. 11 (2015), https://doi.org/10.5334/sta.ez
107. Martić and Đukić, note 18, p. 28.
108. Ibid.
109. Ibid., pp. 28–9.
110. Ibid., p. 29.
111. Ibid.
112. Ibid.
113. Reform Agenda for Bosnia and Herzegovina 2015–2018 (Working Translation) [hereinafter Reform Agenda for BiH], http://europa.ba/wp-content/uploads/2015/09/Reform-Agenda-BiH.pdf. (accessed July 22, 2019), ¶ 8.
114. Martić and Đukić, note 22, p. 29. As Martić and Đukić elaborate, if consumption taxes, such as excise duties on luxury or VAT, covered a great part of health expenses, healthcare financing would be more progressive in the sense that the wealthier segment of the population who consumes more would pay more. The result is even better (in terms of bringing in more money) if the goods taxed are direct expenses, such as taxes on property and profit. Ibid.
115. See generally Vesna Bojicic-Dzelilovic, note 106.
116. This chapter ("Unveiling the Four Hallmarks," past paragraph).
117. Chan, note 12, pp. vi, vii.
118. See Martić and Đukić, note 22, p.26.

119. World Health Organization, *The World Health Report 2000*, note 3, p. 144.
120. Ibid.
121. "The World Health Organization's Ranking of the World's Health Systems, by Rank," *Countries of the World*, photius.com/rankings/healthranks.html

# PART III

# Toward Preventive Medicine in Bosnia

# CHAPTER 5

# Defining Genetic Counseling

**Abstract** This chapter defines genetic counseling, a key term in the book, including an explanation of genetic disorder and the role of the genetic counselor in genetic counseling.

**Keywords** Genetic disorders • Genetic counselor • Genetic counseling

The Chinese thinker Confucius (551–479) once famously stated that the beginning of wisdom is to call things by their proper names. Confucius elaborated that social disorder stemmed from a failure to call things by their right names.[1] A concept so central to the message of this book needing to be called by its proper name is genetic counseling. This chapter fills that bill, in obedience to Confucius's admonition.

## Genetic Disorder

Because *genetic counselors* are workers who provide counseling related to genetic disorders, to define *genetic counseling*, it is necessary to first explain *genetic disorder*. A genetic disorder is a disease condition that is caused by a mutation in an individual's DNA.[2] Genetic disorder may be classified into four major groups: (i) single-gene mutation (which could be dominant, recessive, or x-linked), (ii) multiple-gene mutation, (iii) chromosomal changes (i.e., entire areas of the chromosome can be miss-ing or misplaced), and (iv) mitochondrial mutations (which occur when the maternal genetic material in mitochondria mutate as well).[3]

"There are over 600 genetic disorders, many of which are fatal or severely debilitating."[4] Every year, nearly 8 million infants worldwide, comprising 6% of all births, are born with serious birth disorders.[5] Of this number, an estimated 3.2 million infants, representing over 40%, become disabled for life.[6] Before 2003, the genes associated with many genetic disorders were unknown.[7] The situation changed in 2003 with the com-pletion of the Human Genome Project.[8] Since then, scientists have devel-oped genetic testing that can confirm a diagnosis or a carrier state of the disease, or predict future illness and responses to therapy.[9] Today, over 2000 genetic tests are available.[10] Table 5.1 contains a list of ten most common genetic disorders.[11] Although only six out of the ten are ranked significant in prevalence for Bosnia, this is huge enough for a small, resource-poor country still reeling from the effects of a bloody war years ago that destroyed nearly one-third of its healthcare infrastructure.[12] Instructively, a WHO report on disability published in 2011 found that the extra cost of living with disability in BiH was 14%.[13] In practical terms, this means that in the country, children aged eleven to fifteen years whose parents experienced health problems were 14% more likely than other chil-dren in that age group to drop out of school.[14]

## GENETIC COUNSELING AND THE GENETIC COUNSELOR

"Genetic counseling is a process designed to evaluate and understand a family's risk of an inherited medical condition,"[15] to help affected indi-viduals make responsible and informed decisions about their own health or their child's.[16] During this process, a genetic counselor meets with indi-viduals afflicted with a genetic disorder or at risk of passing on an inherited disorder, whether pregnant women, infants, or adults. The goal is to mini-mize the chances that sufferers or suspected sufferers will transmit the disorder to their offspring, but it is also to support individuals in the deci-sions they make.[17] Genetic counseling traditionally occurs in-person, but it may also occur via alternative methods like a telephone call or group counseling.[18] In this book, the term "genetic counseling" refers to tradi-tional in-person counseling.[19]

Consistent with the Convention on Human Rights and Biomedicine, "genetic counseling" is a "communication process,"[20] which precedes

**Table 5.1**  Ten most common genetic disorders subject to genetic testing and counseling, including the extent of their prevalence in Bosnia

| Item No. | Name of disorder | Description and characteristic symptoms | Prevalence in Bosnia |
|---|---|---|---|
| 1. | Cystic Fibrosis | An autosomal recessive chronic disorder that causes sufferers to produce thick and sticky mucus, inhibiting their respiratory, digestive, and reproductive systems[a] | Significant, rather than negligible[b] |
| 2. | Down's Syndrome (also known as Trisomy 21) | A chromosomal disorder caused by the presence of all or part of a third copy of chromosome 21. Symptoms include delays in physical growth, characteristic facial features, and mild to moderate intellectual disability[c] | Significant, rather than negligible[d] |
| 3. | Fragile X Syndrome | A dominant disorder, linked to the X chromosome, which causes a range of developmental problems, including cognitive impairment and learning disabilities. Sufferers usually have delayed speech and language development by age two. Males are often more severely affected by this disorder[e] | Probably significant[f] |
| 4. | Hemophilia | A bleeding disorder, linked to the X chromosome, which affects the body's ability to produce blood clots. Symptoms include easy bruising, longer bleeding after an injury, and increased risk of bleeding inside joints or the brain[g] | Probably insignificant[h] |
| 5. | Huntington | An autosomal dominant disorder that causes certain nerve cells in the brain and the central nervous system to degenerate. It starts between the thirty- to fifty-year age range and leads to death fifteen to twenty years later[i] | Probably significant[j] |
| 6. | Duchenne Muscular Dystrophy (DMD) | A recessive genetic disorder, linked to the X chromosome, characterized by progressive muscle degeneration and weakness. It is caused by an absence of dystrophin, a protein that helps keep muscle cells intact, and usually leads to death in the early teen years[k] | Probably insignificant[l] |
| 7. | Sickle Cell Anemia | An autosomal recessive disorder that is caused by abnormal hemoglobin, which results in distorted (sickled) red blood cells. Sickled red blood cells are fragile and prone to rupture, which leads to anemia, pain, delays in growth, and frequent infections[m] | Probably significant[n] |

(continued)

**Table 5.1**    (continued)

| Item No. | Name of disorder | Description and characteristic symptoms | Prevalence in Bosnia |
|---|---|---|---|
| 8. | Thalassemia | An autosomal recessive disorder which is caused by abnormal hemoglobin and results in the destruction of red blood cells. Symptoms include anemia, fatigue, deformities of facial bones, delays in growth, and pale appearance[o] | Probably insignificant[p] |
| 9. | Tay-Sachs | An autosomal recessive disorder which affects both sexes equally and results in the destruction of nerve cells in the brain and spinal cord[q] | Probably insignificant[r] |
| 10. | Angelman Syndrome | A rare neurogenetic disorder which affects both sexes equally. Symptoms include delayed development, intellectual disability, severe speech impairment, and epilepsy. Persons with this condition require continuous care and are unable to live independently[s] | Probably significant[t] |

See notes a–t below and accompanying texts

[a]See ARUP Laboratories, Cystic Fibrosis Carrier Testing: What You Need to Know (July 2016), https://www.aruplab.com/files/resources/branding/Brochure_patient_cystic.pdf

[b]See ibid. A person's chance of being a carrier of this condition depends on that person's ethnicity. *Id.* The percentage of Caucasians living with this condition is 92%, topped only by Askenazi Jews at 96%. Ibid. Since Bosnians typically are classified as Caucasians, the prevalence of the condition in the country is not negligible. See also World Health Org., *The Molecular Genetic Epidemiology of Cystic Fibrosis*, https://www.who.int/genomics/publications/en/HGN_WB_04.02_fig 2.pdf

[c]See Amina Kurtovic-Kozaric et al., "Ten-Year Trends in Prevalence of Down Syndrome in a Developing Country: Impact of the Maternal Age and Prenatal Screening," *Eur. J. Obstetrics & Gynecology and Reprod. Biology*, 206 (2016), 79, https://www.ejog.org/article/S0301-2115(16)30894-6/pdf

[d]See ibid. Down's syndrome is one of the most common birth defects that affect about 1 of every 750–1100 live births. Ibid., p. 82. A study published in 2016 found that "[t]he calculated incidence for the live born T21 individuals in Bosnia [was] 1:999. The live-birth prevalence of T21 was 9.6 per 10,000 births and the total prevalence of T21 was 19.1." Ibid., p. 79

[e]Jennifer A. Jewell, "Fragile X Syndrome," *Medscape*, https://emedicine.medscape.com/article/943776-overview, *archived at* https://perma.cc/96AL-RZ78

[f]See ibid. Worldwide, fragile X syndrome is believed to be the most common cause of inherited mental retardation, intellectual disability, and autism, as well as the second most common cause of genetically associated mental deficiencies, second only to Down's syndrome. Ibid. "Fragile X Syndrome affects approximately 1 in 2,500–4,000 males and 1 in 7,000–8,000 females. The prevalence of female carrier status has been estimated to be [about] 1 in 130–250 [persons]; the prevalence of male carrier status is estimated to be [about] 1 in 250–800 [persons]." Ibid.

[g]"What Is Hemophilia?," Centers for Disease Control and Prevention, https://www.cdc.gov/ncbddd/

*(continued)*

**Table 5.1** (continued)

hemophilia/facts.html, *archived at* https://perma.cc/XX7U-FYM5

[h]See World Fed'n of Hemophilia, *Report on the Annual Global Survey* (Dec. 2011), 12, https://www1. wfh.org/publication/files/pdf-1427.pdf. With a population indicated as 4.6 million in 2010, BiH reported 140 people living with hemophilia. *Id.* Emphasis on "probably" is advised because the data BiH provided was for 2006 and given the tentativeness of the report, which cautioned that "[a]ll data are provisional." Ibid. (inside the front page of the document preceding the table of contents)

[i]Šejma Beganović et al., *Huntington's Disease-Case Report* (2015), 48, http://gyrus.hiim.hr/images/ suplement2/neuro2015_Part24.pdf

[j]See ibid. (noting that as of 2015, 8–10 per 100,000 inhabitants in the world live with this condition, compared to 4.46 per 100,000 inhabitants in BiH)

[k]"Rare Disease Database: Duchenne Muscular Dystrophy," Nat'l Org. for Rare Disorders, https://rare-diseases.org/rare-diseases/duchenne-muscular-dystrophy/, *archived at* https://perma.cc/S38A-8U4W (the database is updated periodically with the last being in 2016)

[l]DMD ranks as the most common childhood onset form of muscular dystrophy and mostly affects males, compared to girls. The worldwide numbers are about 1 in every 3500 male births, compared to about 1 in 50 million girls. Ibid.; "Girls Living with Duchenne," Duchenne UK (2019), https://www.duchenneuk. org/girls-living-with-duchenne, *archived at* https://perma.cc/929Z-EFYN. Given its status as "a rare genetic disease affecting only a small percentage of the population," the prevalence of DMD in BiH is assessed as probably insignificant. "Duchenne Muscular Dystrophy | Niche and Rare Pharmacor | G7 | 2015," *DRG* (Dec. 2015), https://decisionresourcesgroup.com/report/141434-biopharma-duchenne-muscular-dystrophy-niche-and-rare/, *archived at* https://perma.cc/SJP6-N58E

[m]See "Sickle Cell Anemia," Mayo Clinic, https://www.mayoclinic.org/diseases-conditions/sickle-cell-anemia/symptoms-causes/syc-20355876, *archived at* https://perma.cc/A3FJ-LHVE

[n]See World Health Org., *The Global Prevalence of Anaemia in 2011* (2015), 19 tbl.A3.1 (ranking BiH "moderate" in-between "severe" and "mild" in 2011 in a table for "Country estimates for children aged 6–59 months"). However, prevalence of the condition is assessed as probably significant for BiH because, although sickle cell trait affects African Americans disproportionately (about 8–10% of the estimated more than 100 million people worldwide with sickle cell trait), "[s]ickle cell trait can also affect Hispanics, South Asians, Caucasians from southern Europe, and people from Middle Eastern countries." See *Frequently Asked Questions Regarding Sickle Cell Trait*, Am. Soc'y of Hematology, https://www.hematology.org/ advocacy/policy-statements/2012/faq-regarding-sickle-cell-trait, *archived at* https://perma. cc/9BFX-HQ5U

[o]"Thalassemia," Mayo Clinic, https://www.mayoclinic.org/diseases-conditions/thalassemia/symptoms-causes/syc-20354995, *archived at* https://perma.cc/4S2A-QMC4

[p]See Tayebeh Noori et al., "International Comparison of Thalassemia Registries: Challenges and Opportunities," *Acta Informatica Medica* [*J. of Acad. of Med. Sciences of Bosn. & Herz.*], 27(1) (Mar. 2019), 58, https://www.ncbi.nlm.nih.gov/pmc/articles/PMC6511274/. The World Health Organization estimates the frequency of carriers of thalassemia and abnormal hemoglobin to be about "5.1% with nearly 226 million carriers worldwide." Ibid., p. 58. Of this number, nearly 80% of thalassemia cases "are detected in the area extending from sub-Saharan Africa to the Mediterranean Basin, the Middle East, and South and Southeast Asia." Ibid.

[q]"Rare Disease Database: Tay Sachs Disease," Nat'l Org. for Rare Disorders, https://rarediseases.org/ rare-diseases/tay-sachs-disease/, *archived at* https://perma.cc/6334-28JR (the database is updated periodically with the last being in 2017)

*(continued)*

**Table 5.1** (continued)

<sup>r</sup>The basis for the indicated assessment is because this disease is a rare condition more frequent among Jewish people of Ashkenazi descent, with approximately 1 in 30 carrying the altered gene for the disease, compared to about "[1] in 300 individuals of non-Ashkenazi Jewish heritage." The number translates into about 1 in 3600 live births. Ibid.

<sup>s</sup>See "Rare Disease Database: Angelman Syndrome," Nat'l Org. for Rare Disorders, https://rarediseases. org/rare-diseases/angelman-syndrome/, *archived at* https://perma.cc/RTB8-N7K3 (the database is updated periodically with the last being in 2018)

<sup>t</sup>*Compare* ibid. (disclosing that the prevalence of this disease is about 1 in 12,000–20,000 people in the general population, although many cases go undiagnosed, which makes it difficult to determine the actual prevalence within the population), *with* Amina Kurtovic-Kozaric et al., "Diagnostics of Common Microdeletion Syndromes Using Fluorescence in situ Hybridization: Single Center Experience in a Developing Country," *Bosn. J. Basic Med. Sci.*, 16(2) (2016), 121, https://www.bjbms.org/ojs/index. php/bjbms/article/view/994/263 (finding for BiH a higher incidence than the rest of Europe from their analysis of a set of microdeletion syndromes, including Angelman syndrome). Parallel to the National Organization for Rare Disorders (NORD), the study "emphasize[d] that the microdeletion syndromes are in general underdiagnosed," leading these investigators to caution that the results they unearthed "can serve as a preliminary basis for creating future guidelines for pediatric genetic diagnosis." Ibid., p. 125. The study (and therefore its results) focused only on one entity, the Federation of Bosnia and Herzegovina, rather than all of BiH

genetic testing.[21] Individuals respond differently to genetic test results[22]; thus, to obtain individuals' informed consent, it is necessary to provide proper counseling by qualified genetic counselors who can help individuals understand the meaning and significance of their test results.[23] The Additional Protocol to the Convention on Human Rights and Biomedicine requires genetic testing for health purposes to be conducted under individualized medical supervision, accompanied by genetic counseling.[24] The treaty sets forth principles related to the quality of genetic services and genetic counseling. One such requirement is that tests predictive of genetic diseases should include appropriate counseling to minimize patients' misunderstanding of the test results and patients' potential anxiety and legitimate related concerns.[25] These concerns include embarrassment, discrimination, and stigmatization, if genetic information is improperly disclosed.[26]

The genetic counselor, "a health professional with specialized training in medical genetics and counseling," is a central figure in genetic counseling.[27] General counselors help persons with genetic disorders (as explained above) and their families. They work in several areas of healthcare, including hospitals, doctor's offices, genetic testing laboratories, research outfits, public health, and insurance companies.[28] Four clinical settings in which genetic counselors practice their wares are prenatal, pediatric, adult, and cancer.[29]

In the *prenatal setting*, women or couples who are pregnant or planning to become pregnant may see a prenatal genetic counselor for reasons that include personal or family history of a known or suspected condition; advanced maternal or paternal age, as the chances for chromosome abnormalities, such as Down's syndrome or single gene disorders increase with parental age; and exposures during pregnancy which may cause birth defects.[30] In the *pediatric setting*, genetic counseling is appropriate for children with conditions, such as a family history of a genetic disorder or suspected genetic disorder, developmental delay, autism spectrum disorders, multiple health problems or birth defects, and abnormal physical features.[31] Establishing an underlying genetic cause for these problems can provide information to affected family members on what to expect in the future, prognosis of the condition, chances of having additional children, and access to support groups and services.[32]

In the *adult setting*, individuals with a personal or family history or symptoms of an adult-onset genetic condition may benefit from genetic counseling to learn about: the risk that they or their children may be diagnosed with or develop an adult-onset condition, and genetic testing options available for diagnosis or predictive testing.[33] In the *cancer setting*, genetic counselors can help persons determine whether or not they have inherited an increased risk for cancer.[34] Under this last category, persons who see a general counselor include individuals with a personal or family history of cancer.[35]

This chapter is the first of three conversations tied to the theme of preventive medicine that drives this book. The next logical step in the progression, to which this book turns, is Chap. 6, which lays out the status of genetic counseling in Bosnia. This analysis is a prelude to Chap. 7 on strategies for promoting preventive medicine through genetic counseling, the main course of this book, to use a food analogy.

## NOTES

1. See James Legge, *Confucian Analects, The Great Learning, and the Doctrine of the Mean* (Mineola, N.Y.: Dover Publications, 1971), 263–64 (translating Analects, Book XIII, Chap. 3, verses 4–7).
2. The acronym is shorthand for deoxyribonucleic acid, the hereditary material in humans and almost all other organisms. See "What is DNA," *Genetics Home Reference* (US National Library of Medicine), https://ghr.nlm.nih.gov/primer/basics/dna

3. Liat Ben-Senior, "10 Most Common Genetic Diseases," *LabRoots* (May 22, 2018), labroots.com/trending/infographics/8833/10-common-genetic-diseases

4. Ibid.

5. Ingrid Lobo & Kira Zhaurova, "Birth Defects: Causes and Statistics," *Nature Educ.* 1(1) (2008), 18, https://www.nature.com/scitable/top-icpage/birth-defects-causes-and-statistics-863/

6. Ibid.

7. See "History of the Human Genome Project," *Human Genome Project Info. Archive 1990–2003,* https://web.ornl.gov/sci/techresources/Human_Genome/project/hgp.shtml, *archived at* https://perma.cc/E5P8-EFEQ (referring to the international thirteen-year effort from 1990 to 2003 "to discover all the estimated 20,000–25,000 human genes and make them accessible for further biological study"); see also "Human Genome Project FAQ," *Nat'l Human Genome Research Inst.*, https://www.genome.gov/human-genome-project/Completion-FAQ, *archived at* https://perma.cc/8BLR-VLDK

8. Ibid. See also Victor K. McElheny, *Drawing the Map of Life: Inside the Human Genome Project* (Basic Books, 2010); Robert Krulwich, "Cracking the Code of Life," PBS Television Show (2003), pbs.org.wgbh/nova/genome/

9. See notes 7–8; see also M.M. Gottesmann & F.S. Collins, Symposium, "The Role of the Human Genome Project in Disease Prevention," *Preventive Med.*, 23(5) (1994), 591.

10. Ben-Senior, note 3; see also Kathryn A. Phillips et al., "Genetic Test Availability and Spending: Where Are We Now? Where Are We Going?," *Health Aff.*, 37(5) (May 2018), 710 ("As of August 1, 2017, there were approximately 75,000 genetic tests on the market, representing approximately 10,000 unique test types.").

11. Ben-Senior, note 3.

12. Jennifer Cain et al., eds., *Health Care Systems in Transition: Bosnia and Herzegovina* (Copenhagen: European Observatory on Health Care Systems, 2002), 17 (putting the size of damage as 30%).

13. World Health Organization, *World Report on Disability* (Geneva, Switzerland: World Health Organization, 2011), 40, 43, 271–80 (Technical Appendix A titled "Estimates of Disability Prevalence (%) and Years of Health Lost Due to Disability (YLD), By Country"), who.int/disabilities/world_report/2011/report.pdf.

14. Ibid., p. 142.

15. "About Genetic Counselors: Genetic Counseling Prospective Student Frequently Asked Questions," Nat'l Soc'y of Genetic Counselors, https://www.nsgc.org/page/frequently-asked-questions-students, archived at https://perma.cc/KN2E-32Q2 [hereinafter About Genetic Counselors].

16. Caroline Bowditch, "Genetic Counseling," *Encyclopedia Britannica*, https://www.britannica.com/science/genetic-counselling, *archived at* https://perma.cc/HR8G-KTSJ

17. Ibid.

18. Jeanna M. McCuaig et al., "Next Generation Service Delivery: A Scoping Review of Patient Outcomes Associated with Alternative Models of Genetic Counseling and Genetic Testing for Hereditary Cancer," *Cancers (Basel)*, 10(11) (2018), 435.

19. See generally ibid. (noting that, compared to alternative methods, traditional in-person genetic counseling is linked with higher acceptance of genetic testing and patient satisfaction).

20. Louiza Kalokairinou et al., "Legislation of Direct-to-Consumer Genetic Testing in Europe: A Fragmented Regulatory Landscape," *J. Cmty. Genetics*, 9(2) (2018), 117, 122. ("[G]enetic counselling is a communication process aiming to support patients in taking informed healthcare decisions, after understanding the benefits, limitations and implications of a genetic test for themselves and their family and being informed about available healthcare options."). See also Elina Rantanen, Expectations, Frames[,] and Practices of Genetic Counselling in Different Contexts of Genetic Testing, Ph.D. dissert., Univ. of Turku (Finland, 2014), 9–10, https://www.utupub.fi/bitstream/handle/10024/98897/Annales%20D%201130%20Rantanen%20DISS.pdf?sequence=2&isAllowed=y.(stating similarly)

21. See Convention for the Protection of Human Rights and Dignity of the Human Being with Regard to the Application of Biology and Medicine: Convention on Human Rights and Biomedicine, Art. 12, January 12, 1999, E.T.S. No. 164 ("Tests which are predictive of genetic diseases or which serve either to identify the subject as a carrier of a gene responsible for a disease or to detect a genetic predisposition or susceptibility to a disease may be performed only for health purposes or for scientific research linked to health purposes, and *subject to appropriate genetic counselling*.") (emphasis added); see also Kalokairinou et al., note 20 (discussing countries where genetic counseling is required or recognized as a necessity before conducting genetic tests, after, or both).

22. See Heidi Carment Howard & Pascal Borry, "Survey of European Clinical Geneticists on Awareness, Experiences and Attitudes toward Direct-to-Consumer Genetic Testing," *Genome Med.*, 5(5) (2013), 45.

23. Kalokairinou et al., note 20, p. 127 ("[I]t may be argued that, in the context of genetic testing, unless genetic counselling takes place, consent cannot really be informed.").

24. Additional Protocol to the Convention on Human Rights and Biomedicine, Concerning Biomedical Research, January 9, 2007, C.E.T.S. No. 195. See

also Laurence Lwoff, "Council of Europe Adopts Protocol on Genetic Testing for Health Purposes," *Eur. J. Hum. Genetics*, 17(11) (July 2009), 1374.

25. See notes 23–4.

26. Kyle B. Brothers & Mark A. Rothstein, "Ethical, Legal and Social Implications of Incorporating Personalized Medicine into Healthcare," *Personalized Med.*, 12(1) (2015), 43, 44.

27. "About Genetic Counselors," note 15, p. 4. In the United States, becoming a genetic counselor requires completion of a master's degree at an accredited genetic counseling program. These programs include rigorous didactic coursework, clinical training, and some research. After completing this training, graduates must pass a board examination to become certified as genetic counselors. Some states require genetic counselors to have a professional license to practice in that state, and the number of states with this requirement appears to be growing. Ibid., p. 1.

28. "About Genetic Counselors," note 15, p. 4.

29. Ibid.

30. Ibid.

31. Ibid.

32. Ibid.

33. Ibid.

34. Ibid.

35. Ibid. This includes cancer in those under the age of fifty, such as breast or colon cancer, two or more first-degree relatives on the same side of their family who have been diagnosed with cancer, more than one primary cancer in the same individual, more than one type of cancer in the same individual, a rare type of cancer or tumor pathology, a known genetic mutation in a cancer susceptibility gene in their family, and an ethnicity associated with a higher frequency of hereditary cancer syndromes. Ibid.

# CHAPTER 6

# Status of Genetic Counseling in the Bosnian Healthcare System

**Abstract** This chapter gauges the status of genetic counseling in the Bosnian healthcare system, the main technique of preventive medicine at the heart of this book. It is a two-part presentation that analyzes the ranking of Bosnia in a multination European survey on the state of the field in 2005–2006 and events since then.

**Keywords** Direct-to-consumer (DTC) genetic tests

This book will be incomplete without gauging the status of genetic counseling in the Bosnian healthcare system, the main technique of preventive medicine at the cynosure of this work. This section fills that gap. However, from an evidentiary standpoint that determination on status is hard to make because of many still moving parts related to genetic counseling in Bosnia and Herzegovina twenty-five years after the war, complicated by inadequate data. Accordingly, this presentation is a portraiture in two parts: BiH's ranking among European countries on a survey in 2005–2006 as starting point; and genetic counseling events in the aftermath of the survey, including three recent developments.

## BOSNIA'S RANK IN A SURVEY ON GENETIC COUNSELING IN 2005–2006

Since the 1960s, European physicians and other medical personnel have provided genetic tests to their patients for health-related reasons within a clinical setting. These tests are usually preceded by a "medical referral, genetic counselling, and [...] informed consent."[1] In contrast, genetic counseling in BiH is suboptimal. This suboptimal level mirrors the overall condition of the healthcare system, which includes genetic counseling. In 2005, EuroGentest, an agency of the European Commission,[2] sponsored a study published in 2006, which surveyed attitudes toward regulations and practices on genetic counseling in thirty-eight European countries, including BiH. The survey tapped the views of countries indirectly through their national representatives, using the EuroGentest network in the country in question, such as the National Society of Human Genetics (NSHG), or the European Society of Human Genetics (ESHG).[3]

The survey revealed the following: of five questions, respondents from BiH answered yes to only one question[4]—whether it would be necessary or good to regulate practical work.[5] Notice that this is an affirmative answer that sounds very much like a negative because it mirrors the remaining answers: the respondents thought it would be a good idea to regulate practical work on genetic counseling because no such regulation at the time existed. On the remaining four questions, the same Bosnian respondents responded in the negative: no on the existence of legislation,[6] no on professional guidelines,[7] no on generally applied practices related to genetic counseling,[8] and no to a "generally applied practice of informed consent."[9] The Bosnian respondents also reportedly answered that the country's genetic counseling could not be viewed as organized.[10] Regarding predictions of future development relating to genetic counseling, the respondents foresaw only "[d]evelopment through [the] private sector."[11] The relative lack of legislation in genetic counseling in Bosnia can be attributed to the newness of genetic testing and counseling. Whatever the reason, the paucity is paradoxical, given the nature of Bosnia and Herzegovina, rooted in its socialist past, as a rule-bound and bureaucratic society.[12]

## GENETIC COUNSELING EVENTS SINCE 2006

Since the 2005–2006 survey, reckonable changes bordering on genetic testing and counseling have taken place in the Bosnian healthcare system. The first relates to laws. For example, all thirteen units that make up the Bosnian healthcare system now have their own healthcare and health insurance laws.[13] While these laws help protect patients' privacy, preserve their dignity, and keep their data confidential,[14] none of the legislation directly addresses genetic counseling. Instead, to take genetic testing, a process inseparable from genetic counseling, as recently as 2012, growth in this field remained at the infancy stage with clinical testing limited to three purposes: "diagnostic[s], research, and basic human genetic research."[15] Inescapably, the limited progress includes laws and their metamorphosis into agency regulations to guide clinical practice.[16]

Another key development relates to the evolution of genetic testing centers across BiH, such as "the Clinical Center of the University of Sarajevo, the Institute for Genetic Engineering and Biotechnology at the University of Sarajevo, the University Clinical Center in Banja Luka, and the University Clinical Center in Tuzla."[17] Genetic tests are available to patients through physician referral and cover areas like prenatal DNA characterization, breast cancer risk, thrombophilia, and genotyping the spectrum of inherited disorders.[18] But because genetic counseling services are available for only a few rare diseases, current efforts in BiH laboratories have focused on advancing physicians' knowledge and professional skills in preventing and diagnosing rare diseases early on.[19] There has also been a focus on "increasing the number of highly specialized personnel" in clinical genetics.[20] Additionally, because Bosnia and Herzegovina lacks certified genetic laboratories for complex diagnostic testing, the few that exist collaborate with certified laboratories outside the country.[21]

A third recent development, reinforcing the second, is the emergence of several private labs offering direct-to-consumer (DTC) genetic tests as a way around the formal system.[22] Currently, the public healthcare system is increasingly asked to interpret and counsel on genetic information that has been generated privately or at the clinic.[23] The types of tests these private entities offer vary, including "tests that offer information regarding health enhancement (nutrigenomics, dermato-genetics); drug response (pharmacogenomics); and susceptibility for common complex disorders, [such as] cardiovascular diseases, depression, osteoporosis, [and] type 2 diabetes."[24] Although this commercial phenomenon is making genetic information increasingly available to the general public, it is provided without counseling and people are often unaware that their health risk information is sold.[25] Many DTC genetic testing companies do not provide their consumers with appropriate pre- and post-genetic counseling; however, even when companies provide genetic counseling, concerns arise about the quality and mode of that service.[26] There is also a cost element. While it is important for persons to know their susceptibility risk, the expensive price tag of testing—sometimes more than the average salary of many workers in BiH—makes testing unavailable to many.[27] For this reason, countries should share approaches and draw on lessons learned in disparate locales rather than approach the issue alone.[28]

Finally, not all private companies or labs that offer genetic testing in BiH perform genetic counseling services inside the country. Instead, some of these companies or labs conduct genetic analysis in certified laboratories situated *outside* of the country.[29] Subsequently, they share the test results with the patients and their physicians.[30] In some private companies or labs, certified genetic counselors from companies outside Bosnia, assisted by a translator, advise via Skype.[31] Moreover, the relatively few centers and labs in the country that *have* developed technical and personnel infrastructure to implement more advanced genetic diagnostic services are "not financed from the mandatory health insurance funds."[32] Consequently, the Bosnian population faces difficulties using these service centers.

The status of genetic counseling in BiH tracks the overall condition of the healthcare system of which genetic counseling is part and parcel. This chapter is one of two complementary conversations on steps to promote preventive medicine in Bosnia through genetic counseling. The next, the centerpiece of the discussion, identifies and analyzes the strategies involved in that effort.

## NOTES

1. Louiza Kalokairinou et al., "Legislation of Direct-to-Consumer Genetic Testing in Europe: A Fragmented Regulatory Landscape," *J. Cmty. Genetics*, 9(2) (2018), p. 118. Within the context of genetic testing, medical supervision, genetic counseling, and informed consent are concepts connected to clinical practice, not aspects related to genetic tests as products, such as their clinical validity. These three often overlap in practice. For example, all three have fundamentally similar goals: "to guide users to make decisions about their health based on genetic tests that are appropri-

ate for them, after understanding their benefits, limitations and possible implications." Ibid., pp. 126–27.

2. "What is EuroGentest," *Eur. Society Hum. Genetics* (ESHG), http://www. eurogentest.org/index.php?id=160. Funded by the European Commission, the executive arm of the European Union, this outfit works to harmonize genetic testing in Europe, with a view to ensuring that these tests "provid[e] accurate and reliable results for the benefit of the patients." Ibid.

3. Elina Rantanen et al., Regulations and Practices Related to Genetic Counselling in 38 European Countries, Annex 1 (2006) ("[r]egulations and practices related to genetic counselling in 38 European countries"), www.eurogentest.org/fileadmin/templates/eugt/pdf/Results_of_sur-vey_1_WP_3-1_Dec06.pdf ("Methods")

4. Ibid., p. 11 annex 1 col. 4.

5. Ibid., p. 11 annex 1 col. 4.

6. Ibid., p. 11 annex 1 col. 2.

7. Ibid., p. 11 annex 1 col. 3.

8. Ibid., p. 11 annex 1 col. 5.

9. Ibid., p. 11 annex 1 col. 6.

10. Ibid., p. 11 annex 1 col. 7.

11. Ibid., p. 11 annex 1 col. 8.

12. See, for example, Mladen Lakic, "Bosnian Entrepreneurs Face Bureaucratic Obstacles to Success," *BakanInsight* (Nov. 7, 2018, 7:06 AM), https:// balkaninsight.com/2018/11/07/bosnian-entrepreneurs-struggling-with-administration-amid-creative-ideas-11-06-2018/, *archived at* https://perma.cc/4T8Y-KDXK; Dražen Huterer et al., "Bosnian Divisions Create Bureaucratic Headaches," *Pro.Ba* (2013), https://pro. ba/en/bosnia-divisions-create-bureaucratic-headaches/, *archived at* https://perma.cc/N2BH-MQ97

13. See Sabina Semiz & Philip C. Aka, "Precision Medicine in the Era of CRISPR-Cas9: Evidence from Bosnia and Herzegovina," *Palgrave Communications*, 5 (2019), 1, 3 (discussing the legal and constitutional provisions for healthcare in Bosnia).

14. See Chap. 3 of this book (discussing provisions for healthcare in BiH).

15. See Semiz & Aka, note 13.

16. See ibid., pp. 3–4 ("Genetic testing in Bosnia and Herzegovina" *and* "Genetic counseling in Bosnia and Herzegovina").

17. Ibid., p. 3.

18. Ibid.

19. Ibid.

20. Vladmiri Guzvic et al., "Rare Diseases and Orphan Drugs Accessibility in Bosnia and Herzegovina," *Materia Socio Medica* [*J. of Acad. Of Bosn. & Herz.*], 30(4) (Dec. 2018), 297, 298. The article defines "rare diseases" as

illnesses, such as phenylketonuria and congenital hypothyroidism, which affect less than 1 in 2000 people. Ibid., pp. 297, 299.

21. Semiz & Aka, note 13, p. 3.
22. Pascal Borry et al., "Where Are You Going, Where Have You Been: A Recent History of the Direct-to-Consumer Genetic Testing Market," *J. Cmty. Genetics*, 1(3) (2010), 101. See also Borry et al., Symposium, "Is There a Right Time to Know? The Right Not to Know and Genetic Testing in Children," *J. L. Med., and Ethics*, 42(1) (2014), 19, 20.
23. See Borry et al., note 22, pp. 103–04.
24. Ibid., p. 102.
25. See ibid., p. 103.
26. See Heidi C. Howard & Pascal Borry, "Survey of European Clinical Geneticists on Awareness, Experiences, and Attitudes toward Direct-to-Consumer Genetic Testing," *Genome Med.* 5(5) (2013): 53–4.
27. Semiz & Aka, note 13, p. 4 (citing Vladmiri Guzvic et al., "Health Technology Assessment in Central-Eastern and South Europe Countries: Bosnia and Herzegovina," *Int'l J. Tech. Assessments in Health Care*, 33(3) (2017), 390, 390–95).
28. Teri A. Manolio et al., "Global Implementation of Genomic Medicine: We Are Not Alone," *Sci. Transnat'l. Med.*, 7(290) (2015) ("Abstract"). Transnational collaboration through the large research consortia and sharing information in the areas of health information technology, genomics, pharmacogenomics, education, professional development, and policy and regulatory issues appears to be imperative for the future efficient clinical implementation of personalized medicine at the global level. Ibid. ("Brief Landscape of International Genomic Medicine Projects" and "Opportunities for International Collaboration"). See also Paul Ndebele & Rosemary Musesengwa, "Will Developing Countries Benefit from Their Participation in Genetics Research?" *Malawi Med. J.*, 20(2) (2008), 67 (arguing "for justice in the sharing of both burdens and benefits of genetic research").
29. Semiz & Aka, note 13, p. 4.
30. Ibid.
31. Ibid.
32. Guzvic et al., note 20, p. 300.

# CHAPTER 7

# Implementing Preventive Medicine in Bosnia Through Genetic Counseling

**Abstract** This chapter identifies and discusses several factors all stakeholders may use to implement preventive medicine in Bosnia through genetic counseling. The chapter argues that, for lasting result, genetic counseling as tool of preventive medicine must be backed by progress in alcohol and tobacco controls.

**Keywords** Statutory standards for genetic counseling • Increased public education • Alcohol and smoking controls • Expanding the role of the state-level government in healthcare administration

This chapter identifies and discusses several factors all stakeholders may use to implement preventive medicine in Bosnia through genetic counseling. For lasting result, genetic counseling as tool of preventive medicine must be backed by progress in alcohol and tobacco controls. The applicable stakeholders include political leaders at all levels of government, the public, civil society (or nongovernmental organizations), and international agencies. The means used to pursue that implementation that this chapter analyzes are creating statutory standards for genetic counseling now practically nonexistent, increased public education in genetic counseling, more progress on alcohol and smoking controls, and expanding the role of the state-level government in healthcare administration as a matter of reform.

P. C. Aka, *Genetic Counseling and Preventive Medicine in Post-War Bosnia*, https://doi.org/10.1007/978-981-15-7987-5_7

## CREATING STATUTORY STANDARDS FOR GENETIC COUNSELING NOW PRACTICALLY LACKING

Laws "form[ ] an important framework for practices and services related to genetic testing" and counseling.[1] They "help[ ] to standardize practical work" in the field by guaranteeing "the quality of treatment [...] [for] patients and their families in all medical centers."[2] Furthermore, laws are particularly needed in countries like BiH "where the development of genetic medicine may have been more recent and issues related to human genetics may be a newer area of consideration."[3] Accordingly, for knowledgeable observers, such as the respondents in 2005–2006 survey on genetic counseling commented upon in Chap. 6, the absence of laws "'has a negative impact on practical work in" the field.[4] As indicated in that chapter, particularly the section recounting recent developments relating to the status of genetic counseling in Bosnia, although the country has several laws that relate to healthcare, those are barely sufficient given their tenuous connection to genetic counseling.

Drawing on the 2005–2006 survey, as used here, law combines two concepts: legislation and professional guidelines.[5] *Legislation* "refer[s] to official laws passed by the Parliament [legislative body] and additions that go through a Ministry."[6] Legislation addresses issues like whether a healthcare provider has the requisite training needed for a procedure or activity, such as genetic counseling.[7] *Professional guidelines* refers to "professional and other best practice papers" that are not binding authorities.[8] Professional guidelines may be viewed as rules that "affect counselling even though they do not specifically cover it."[9] A good law in genetic counseling *should* cover clinical situations and topics regarding diagnostic testing, carrier testing, predictive testing, susceptibility testing for multifactorial diseases, prenatal diagnosis, preimplantation diagnosis, testing of children and adolescents, and consent of the patient.[10] A good law should also address the following: who can perform genetic counseling; counseling persons from minority ethnic groups; counseling minors or persons with diminished capacity; providing psychological support during counseling; informing relatives of at-risk patients; matters relating to confidentiality, including circumstances when it is legally permissible to breach confidentiality; nondirectiveness; and the duty to recontact the patient.[11]

Although this is a comprehensive list of topics, the ones most often covered are prenatal diagnosis, informed consent, and confidentiality.[12] Professional guidelines mostly address "counselling in the context of prenatal diagnosis, testing of children and adolescents, non-directiveness of counselling[,] and who can perform genetic counseling."[13] Nonetheless, Bosnia needs a statute that broadly spells out certain guidelines regarding quality control of genetic counseling, one which the health ministry could then flesh out with specific regulations to facilitate implementation. The idea is to create statutory standards for genetic counseling currently practically lacking.

New legislation would signify that an issue in question has made its way successfully to the public policy agenda and is acquiring some level of legitimation there.[14] Creating statutory standards for genetic counseling would also provide indispensable guidelines for administrative agencies, beginning with the Ministry of Health. New legislation does not have to cover all of the topics enumerated in the comprehensive list set forth in the foregoing paragraphs, but, at a minimum, it needs to address the following: parameters of genetic testing, nondiscrimination for individuals with genetic problems, privacy, and confidentiality.[15] Adopting this proposal bearing on the creation of statutory standards for genetic counseling will benefit impoverished people, who, unlike their more materially fortunate compatriots, cannot afford access to good healthcare abroad, such as in the United States, the United Kingdom, Canada, and even neighboring countries in this region with better healthcare systems and access to healthcare services than the ones Bosnia affords.[16]

## INCREASED PUBLIC EDUCATION IN GENETIC COUNSELING

The Council of Europe's directive relating to genetic testing and screening for healthcare sets forth some rules for good practices in genetic testing and screening.[17] These rules include Principle 1 on informing the public.[18] Principle 1 prescribes that "[p]lans [to] introduc[e] [. . .] genetic testing and screening should be brought to the notice of individuals, families[,] and the public."[19] It further provides that "[t]he public should be informed about [. . .] the[] availability, purpose, and implications [of genetic testing and screening, in particular,]" and where they can go to access those services.[20] Principle 1 adds that "[s]uch information should start with the school system and be continued by the media."[21] Recognition of the key role of public education in healthcare dates back at least to the International Conference on Primary Healthcare in September of 1978 at Alma-Ata in the then Soviet Union. The declaration adopted at the conference identified "education concerning prevailing health problems and methods for addressing them" among eight essential elements of primary healthcare.[22]

To accomplish the task of analysis marked out for them, concepts need to be robustly defined. Thus, in the expansive sense it is used here, public engagement is *not* limited to informing and consulting individuals; instead, it also encompasses initiatives designed to educate the public on and foster research of emerging technologies. To ensure ethically reliable and socially acceptable application of new genetic technologies, it is important to recognize the attitudes and concerns of the general public related to these technologies.[23] In a nutshell, increased public education is fundamental for disseminating bioethical principles related to genetic testing and counseling to the BiH public and for promoting widespread application of these new techniques.[24]

Beyond individuals and the public, other stakeholders within society have important complementary roles to play. Patient organizations can advocate for patients at all levels of the government.[25] Here, the associations of health professions should exercise a more active role in organizing continued professional education in Bosnian health centers and clinics on genetic testing and counseling. Universities, including sections of these higher education organizations versed on issues related to genetic counseling and preventive medicine can do the same. If nothing else, such shared role could go a long way in integrating the healthcare system in Bosnia and Herzegovina and improving professional communication across the various health institutions.[26]

Studies show that Bosnian physicians generally lack knowledge related to genetic tests and might not feel competent to interpret their results.[27] Thus, to minimize errors in assessing health risks and to promote disease prevention and treatment options, it is imperative to improve the education of physicians and other health professionals who deal with matters related to genetic counseling. Especially, these professionals should learn about appropriate ways to utilize genetic tests. In addition to point-of-care learning and clinical decision support systems developed to provide physicians with information regarding pharmaco-genetic tests and personalized medicine,[28] there are also opportunities to learn more about genetic testing and counseling through online modules and participatory learning strategies.[29] Furthermore, future Bosnian health professionals should be educated on pharmaco-economics because it will allow them to actively participate in establishing the process for assessing health technology.[30]

One final factor, for this author, bearing on increased public education relates to the lack of university-level education in genetic counseling in Bosnia. The education and professional training required for genetic counselors in Europe are marked by disparities shrouded in varied standards of registration, substance, and duration of instructions and clinical training, down to the existence in some countries of programs in genetic counseling that other countries lack.[31] The European Board of Medical Genetics has recommended that genetic counselors receive a master's degree to meet appropriate academic and professional standards.[32] In considering whether or not to adopt this recommendation, Bosnian authorities may also want to keep in mind that the advice is in harmony with existing practice in the United States.[33]

## MORE PROGRESS ON ALCOHOL AND SMOKING CONTROLS

Due to constraints of space and time, by design, this book focuses mainly on genetic counseling as a tool for preventive medicine in Bosnia, at the virtual expense and relative neglect of equally valid techniques like minimizing alcohol and tobacco abuses. Yet, sustainable progress on genetic counseling must necessarily be joined with progress in tobacco and alcohol controls. There are various other factors more or less impinged on genetic counseling justifying this broadened approach. First, although outside the direct control of the healthcare system, tobacco and alcohol policies affect the health of population.[34] A second factor relates to the emerging evidence on the possible influence of environmental factors embedded in attitudes on genetics.[35] There is a growing awareness today of these environmental forces. Third is the reality that, globally, regulation of tobacco and alcohol uses is "a vital component of the right to health."[36] Finally, from a domestic standpoint, proposals on healthcare reforms in Bosnia, material key to the argument in this book, tend to reference these two issues of public health. For example, the Reform Agenda for Bosnia and Herzegovina 2015–2018 commented on supporting an increase in excise duties on tobacco and alcohol that is then channeled to the insurance funds of all entities, including Brčko District.[37]

Accordingly, assignment of seemingly secondary attention to these two issues in this book is a matter of space and time constraints that must not be read to mean that these matters are not serious. If nothing else, what makes alcohol and tobacco abuses a double whammy for a country that has this problem, especially one like postwar Bosnia faced with the issue is a negative synergy evident in the fact that many heavy smokers combine this habit with excessive alcohol and vice versa, a syndrome some analysts call "concurrent alcohol and tobacco dependence."[38] In 2005, the two ranked among ten leading factors of ill-health and disabilities in the Federation of Bosnia and Herzegovina, the larger of Bosnia's two entities. That said, as indicated in Chap. 1 of this book, and reinforced by Table 7.1, with its list of ten leading risk factors and their disease burdens, isolation of these two controls as object of attention is illustrative; the two are a sample of the numerous issues of public health and environmental protection that Bosnia confronts today.

Unlike smoking (see below), moderate drinking for many is considered socially pleasurable,[39] leaving out excessive drinking as the main issue of concern in this book. Such excessive drinking by definition includes "binge" drinking which takes place when a drinker consumes large

**Table 7.1** Ten leading risk factors and DALYs in FBiH in 2005

| Rank | Men | | Women | |
|------|-----|--|-------|--|
| | Risk factor | Total DALYS (rounded %-age) | Risk factor | Total DALYS (rounded %-age) |
| 1. | Tobacco | 21 | High blood pressure | 14 |
| 2. | High blood pressure | 13 | High BMI | 8 |
| 3. | Alcohol | 9 | Tobacco | 7 |
| 4. | High cholesterol | 7 | High cholesterol | 5 |
| 5. | High BMI | 7 | Physical inactivity | 3 |
| 6. | Low fruit and vegetable | 4 | Low fruit and vegetable | 3 |
| 7. | Physical inactivity | 3 | Unsafe sex | 2 |
| 8. | Illicit drug | 2 | Alcohol | 1 |
| 9. | Lead | 1 | Childhood sexual abuse | 1 |
| 10. | Occupational risk factor and injuries | 1 | Lead | 1 |

Ante Ivankovic et al., "Health Status of Population in Federation of Bosnia and Herzegovina in 15 Years of Transitional Period," *Antropol.* 34 (2010), Supp. 1: 325–27. DALYs, abbreviation for disability-adjusted life years, measures overall disease burden, expressed as the number of years lost due to ill-health, disability, or early death. The measure was developed in the 1990s as a way of comparing the overall health and life expectancy of different countries. See "Metrics: Disability-Adjusted Life Years (DALY)," World Health Org., https://www.who.int/healthinfo/global_burden_disease/metrics_daly/en/

amounts of alcohol within a single session, as opposed to small quantities more frequently.[40] Based on development indicators collected by the World Bank, in 2016, the total alcoholic consumption per capita in Bosnia (i.e., persons fifteen years and above), measured in liters of pure alcohol, comprised of beer, spirits, and wine, was 6.4 liters.[41] That was the global average that year.[42] The quantity can be made more understandable by expressing it in bottles of wine.[43] Wine contains around 12% of pure alcohol per volume; accordingly, 1 liter of wine contains 0.12 liters of pure alcohol. Using this formula of conversion, 6.4 liters of pure alcohol per person per year translates into fifty-three bottles of wine per person fifteen years and above.[44] Yet more simply, 6.4 liters of pure alcohol per person per year equals about 1 liter of wine per week.[45]

Alcohol abuse forms a risk factor for diseases and health-related events like crime, traffic accidents, mental disorder, sexually transmitted diseases (e.g., HIV/AIDS, hepatitis B and C, tuberculosis, and syphilis), and alcohol dependence.[46] In 2016, alcohol and drug abuse disorders contributed nearly 2% of the share of total burden of disease in Bosnia.[47] Some of the estimated 2.8 million premature deaths per year in the world from alcohol consumption are Bosnians.[48] While compared to smoking, discussed below, alcohol abuse might not seem like a big problem in Bosnia, such a conclusion is not true for several reasons. Though it might seem trifle, alcohol abuse in Bosnia is trouble enough for the healthcare system for a country still reeling from the aftereffects of a traumatic war that wreaked havoc on its already-modest healthcare infrastructure. This is especially given the negative synergism between the two habits referred to previously.

Smoking is an endemic problem in BiH.[49] Whereas, by definition, some portion of alcohol is imbued with "pleasure" (see above), it is not the case with smoking, most or all of which is considered to lack redeeming social value. About one of every two adults in the country smokes.[50] The number is up from about one in three in 2012.[51] In 2016, the share of the population ten years and above who smoked daily was approximately 32%.[52] In the same year, the share of the population fifteen years and above who smoked daily was 39%.[53] With a consumption in 2000 of six billion cigarettes, equating to five cigarettes per citizen per day, Bosnians rank among the leading users of cigarettes in Europe.[54]

Tobacco abuse is a leading risk factor for cardiovascular diseases as well as for obstructive and malignant pulmonary diseases.[55] "[N]on-communicable diseases," including those connected to tobacco abuse, "account for 45% of deaths."[56] In 2017, the death rate from smoking was approximately 142.[57] In short, "[t]obacco consumption is a serious health, economic, social, and financial issue for BiH [. . . which] increase[s] diseases, disabilities, and premature deaths, [and places a] financial burden on smokers and their families, health service providers, and employers."[58] What is more, cigarette smoking is sometimes the gateway to psychedelic drugs like LSD, mescaline, PCP, marijuana, and heroin.[59]

In November of 2012, the World Bank organized an international conference on tobacco control held in Sarajevo.[60] The conference was held in partnership with BiH authorities (at both the central and entity levels) and the government of Switzerland.[61] The two-day conference was designed to promote tobacco control in BiH, and to afford a forum for delegates from various countries who attended the conference to share experiences on best practices regarding tobacco control programs.[62] Participants included "key government officials and health specialists from Albania, [BiH], Brazil, Kosovo, Montenegro, Slovenia, Serbia, Turkey, and Ukraine, as well as experts from the World Health Organization, the World Bank, and civil society."[63] At the conference, Mr. Sredoje Nović, then minister of civil affairs, declared, "'[t]he fight against tobacco is one of the key battles that we in Bosnia and Herzegovina have to lead in the period ahead.'"[64] Nonetheless, several years after the conference, smoking remains pervasive in Bosnia.[65] It is estimated that five million people die worldwide as a direct consequence of tobacco smoking and an additional half a million die from second-hand smoke. For a relatively small country, BiH contributes significantly to this death toll.[66]

Over the years, Bosnia has registered some progress related to control of tobacco (ab)uses. These include regulation prohibiting smoking in public places, ban on advertising cigarettes in the mass media as well as on sponsorship by the tobacco industry, increased tax on tobacco products designed to make them less affordable, health warnings on cigarette packages, and a general rise in the awareness on the negative health effects of smoking.[67] However, for various reasons, the progress is barely enough. These include lax enforcement of regulations prohibiting smoking in public places, continued sales of tobacco products to minors (i.e., persons under eighteen years of age), and insufficient number of medical personnel with training in tobacco dependence treatment.[68] In addition, nargile bars are still widespread in Bosnia.[69] Nargile bars are drinking parlors where minors smoke hookah (i.e., "water pipes" in fruit-flavored tobacco).[70] In many jurisdictions, operators of these bars still go unpunished.[71] The addictive propensity and carcinogenic potency of hookah compared to plain cigarettes is still an issue of debate.[72]

The debate needs to include the possible number of minors who graduate into full-flown cigarette smokers from the "minor league" of hookah. Going further, governments at all levels in Bosnia should take control of alcohol and tobacco abuses more seriously by, among other things, implementing more effective enforcement of existing laws and creating new laws to plug detected loopholes. Fortunately, as a starting point, Bosnian law provides treatments for drug addiction.[73]

## EXPANDING THE ROLE OF THE STATE-LEVEL GOVERNMENT IN HEALTHCARE ADMINISTRATION AS A MATTER OF REFORM

One key issue that has been overlooked in the debate on healthcare reforms in Bosnia is the role of the state-level government in healthcare delivery. As indicated in Chap. 1, the healthcare system in Bosnia comprises governmental units in the country, thirteen of them altogether, except the state-level government. There is a need to increase the role of the state-level government in healthcare delivery, to the glory of genetic counseling and preventive medicine. Its participation in crafting the document on Reform Agenda for Bosnia and Herzegovina 2015–2018, analyzed in Chap. 1, speaks to the existence of a role already that the state-level government just needs to expand. By identifying and positioning this lack among the strategies for promoting preventive medicine in Bosnia, this book helps to fill the gap.

Recall the discussion in Chap. 4 on the guide to healthcare reforms in postwar Bosnia and the extent to which the country meets these requirements. With respect to good or more effective laws, under the Constitution of 1995, as well as under the ICESCR of which Bosnia and Herzegovina is a state party, the state-level government has healthcare obligations that it fails to shoulder when it assumes a lackadaisical or lack-luster role in healthcare. By limiting its role to agreements on reform proposals, the state-level government risks abdicating its obligations for healthcare under the Bosnian constitution and international law. Next to good or adequate financing, the state-level government should, at a minimum, increase its contribution to the entities on healthcare. To ensure it does not fight for turf with the powerful entity governments, the central government should make budgetary or donation contributions.

In an era where the theme is on diversifying the sources of healthcare, the central government can come in with (increased) financial support to help what the entities are doing.[74] In 2016, the central government's expenditure as a share of the GDP was over 35%.[75] It would be interesting to know where the money went if none of it went to healthcare. Finally, on good politics, analogized to politics friendly to healthcare, the lapses in the above two hallmarks speak to the failure of politics with respect to healthcare. Still on good politics, increasing its level of participation beyond debate on healthcare reforms demonstrates the preciousness of healthcare of a kind that can help improve funding for healthcare allocation.

This chapter explored strategies for promoting preventive medicine in postwar Bosnia through genetic counseling without glossing over progress in the two public health issues of tobacco and alcohol abuses necessary to solidify that campaign. The ethnic conflict from 1992 to 1995 likely contributed to these public health dilemmas.[76] Instead of surrendering to it, Bosnia and Herzegovina should build on its past by committing to socioeconomic human rights, including healthcare. Bosnia's shortcomings regarding genetic counseling demonstrate the progress that remains to be made. As it struggles to recover from the still-felt effects of the gory conflict that damaged its economy and healthcare system, BiH should implement and promote preventive healthcare, achieved through genetic counseling as well as through progress in public health issues like minimizing alcohol and tobacco abuses.

## NOTES

1. Elina Rantanen et al., Regulations and Practices Related to Genetic Counselling in 38 European Countries, Annex 1 (2006), 2, www.eurogentest.org/fileadmin/templates/eugt/pdf/Results_of_survey_1_WP_3-1_Dec06.pdf
2. Ibid., p. 3 (quoting two respondents).
3. Ibid., p. 4.
4. See ibid.
5. See generally ibid., pp. 2–3 (discussing legislation and guidelines related to genetic testing)
6. Ibid., p. 2.
7. Ibid.
8. Ibid., p. 2.
9. Ibid.
10. See ibid., p. 14 annex 2 (charting "[d]ifferent clinical situations and topics related to genetic counselling in legislation, guidelines and practices of 38 European countries").

11. See ibid. Nondirectiveness, one of the clinical situations and topics enumerated, is present when the geneticist or medical personnel provides genetic information in a balanced fashion, without undue pressure on or coercion of the patient. Typically, this would require providing information that "include[s] the pertinent medical facts, results of tests, [and] the consequences and choices." Additionally, the counselor would "explain the purpose and nature of the tests and point out possible risks." Significantly, these steps are not an exhaustive list of what may be needed to adequately ensure non-directiveness. Council of Europe, Committee of Ministers, Recommendation No. R (92) 3 on Genetic Testing and Screening for Health Care Purposes (February 10, 1992), Principle 3, *reprinted* in *Int'l Digest of Health Legislation*, 43 (1992), 284, http:// hrlibrary.umn.edu/instree/coerecr92-3.html [hereinafter Recommendation No. R (92) 3 on Genetic Testing and Screening for Health Care Purposes].

12. Rantanen et al., note 1, p. 3 (based on information from opinion surveys).

13. Ibid.

14. See "An Introduction to the Public Policy-Making Cycle," *Point Park University Online* (Philadelphia, PA) (posted June 12, 2017), https:// online.pointpark.edu/public-administration/policy-making-cycle/ (focusing on the United States and particularly on Phase 3 on "Policy Legitimation," which is reached when the public views the government's action on the policy matter in question "to be legal and authoritative.").

15. See generally Inst. of Med., Div. of Health Sci. Policy, Comm. on Assessing Genetic Risks, *Assessing Genetic Risks: Implications for Health and Social Policy* (Lori B. Andrews et al. eds., National Academies Press, 1994) (discussing concerns regarding confidentiality, discrimination, and genetic testing in general).

16. This is a practice some critics derisively call "medical tourism." See, for example, Michael D. Horowitz et al., "Medical Tourism: Globalization of the Healthcare Marketplace," *Medscape Gen. Med.*, 9(4) (2007), 33. However, the overall lethargic response of many advanced healthcare systems, including the United States', to the COVID-19 pandemic, see, for example, Jacquelyn Corley, "U.S. Government Response to COVID-19 Was Slow. But How Does It Compare to Other Countries?" *Forbes* (April 10, 2020), https://www.forbes.com/sites/jacquelyncorley/2020/04/ 10/us-government-response-to-covid-19-was-slow-but-how-does-it-compare-to-other-countries/, puts a big question mark on the perceived benefits of medical tourism.

17. See generally Recommendation No. R(92) 3 on Genetic Testing and Screening for Health Care Purposes, note 11.

18. Ibid., principle 1.

19. Ibid., principle 1(a).
20. Ibid., principle 1(b).
21. Ibid.
22. World Health Organization, *World Health Report 1995: Bridging the Gaps* (Geneva: World Health Organization), 88 (Box 18), https://www.who.int/whr/1995/en/whr95_en.pdf?ua=1
23. Davit Chokoshvili et al., "Public Views on Genetics and Genetic Testing: A Survey of the General Public in Belgium," *Genetic Testing and Molecular Biomarkers*, 21(3) (2017), 195–201 (focusing on Belgium).
24. Lejla Mahmutović et al., "Perceptions of Students in Health and Molecular Life Sciences Regarding Pharmacogenomics and Personalized Medicine, ' *Human Genomics*, 12(1) (2018), 50 ("Conclusions").
25. Vladmiri Guzvic et al., "Rare Diseases and Orphan Drugs Accessibility in Bosnia and Herzegovina," *Materia Socio Medica [J. of Acad. Of Bosn. & Herz.]*, 30(4) (Dec. 2018), 297, 298. See also Lynn G. Dressler et al., "Genomics Education for the Public: Perspectives of Genomic Researchers and ELSI Advisors," *Genetic Testing and Molecular Biomarkers*, 18(3) (2014), 131, 138 (suggesting that roundtable discussions, expert discussions, workshops, and symposia are needed to bring together key interdisciplinary stakeholders in academia, government, profit, and nonprofit organizations to create programs for the public dealing with genetic education).
26. See Ahmed Novo et al., "Measures to Improve Integration of Healthcare in Federation of Bosnia and Herzegovina," *Materia Socio Medica [J. of Acad. of Med. Sciences of Bosn. & Herz.]*, 31(1) (2019), 71 (focusing on FBiH rather than on the whole country).
27. See Diane Hauser et al., "Views of Primary Care Providers on Testing Patients for Genetic Risks for Common Chronic Diseases," *Health Aff.*, 37(5) (2018), 793, 794.
28. See, for example, Peter H. O'Donnell et al., "Pharmacogenomics-Based Point-of-Care Clinical Decision Support Significantly Alters Drug Prescribing," *Clinical Pharmacology & Therapeutics*, 102(5) (2017), 859.
29. Susanne B. Haga et al., "Primary Care Physicians' Knowledge, Attitudes, and Experience with Personal Genetic Testing," *J. of Pers. Med.*, 9(2) (2019), 29, 37–38.
30. See Tarik Catic & Selma Skrbo, "Pharmaco-economic Education for Pharmacy Students in Bosnia and Herzegovina," *Materia Socio Medica [J. of Acad. of Med. Sciences of Bosn. & Herz.]*, 25(4) (2013), 282, 282–83.
31. See generally Milena Paneque et al., "Development of a Registration System for Genetic Counsellors and Nurses in Health-care Services in Europe," *Eur. J. Hum. Genetics*, 24 (2016), 312 (discussing the start of the

genetic counseling profession and the attempt by the European Board of Medical Genetics to build a registration system for professionals, with a brief overview of that system's progress).

32. Ibid., p. 312.

33. "About Genetic Counselors: Genetic Counseling Prospective Student Frequently Asked Questions," National Society of Genetic Counselors, https://www.nsgc.org/page/frequently-asked-questions-students, archived at https://perma.cc/KN2E-32Q2 (noting that in the United States, genetic counselors are required to complete a master's degree at an accredited genetic counseling program).

34. Marina Karanikolos et al., "Comparing Population Health," *in* Irene Papanicolas & Peter C. Smith, eds., *Health System Comparison: An Agenda for Policy, Information and Research* (Maidenhead, UK: Open University Press, 2013), 128.

35. See, for example, Kendra Cherry, "The Age Old Debate of Nature vs. Nurture," *VeryWellMind* (updated September 4, 2019), https://www.verywellmind.com/what-is-nature-versus-nurture-2795392; and Ingrid Lobo, "Environmental Influences on Gene Expression," *Nature Educ.*, 1(1) 39 (2008), 39, https://www.nature.com/scitable/topicpage/environmental-influences-on-gene-expression-536/

36. See Oscar A. Cabrera & Lawrence O. Gostin, "Global Tobacco Control: A Vital Component of the Right to Health," *in* José M. Zuniga et al., eds., *Advancing the Human Right to Health* (New York: Oxford Univ. Press, 2013), 261–74 (focusing on tobacco control).

37. Reform Agenda for Bosnia and Herzegovina 2015–2018 (Working Translation). http://europa.ba/wp-content/uploads/2015/09/Reform-Agenda-BiH.pdf, archived at https://perma.cc/X385-JW5K

38. See David J. Drobes, "Concurrent Alcohol and Tobacco Dependence," Nat'l Inst. on Alcohol Abuse and Alcoholism (Nov. 2002), https://pubs.niaaa.nih.gov/publications/arh26-2/136-142.htm

39. See Hannah Ritchie & Max Roser, "Alcohol Consumption," *Our World in Data* (April 2018, updated November 2019), https://ourworldindata.org/alcohol-consumption (first paragraph of article). See also Lejla Bečar, "Alcoholism: The Socially Acceptable Disease," *Balkan Diskurs* (July 26, 2015), https://balkandiskurs.com/en/2015/26/alcoholism-the-socially-acceptable-disease/ (though what this article meant was alcohol consumed moderately, rather than excessively); and Sam Bedford, "[Eleven] Reasons Why Drinking in Bosnia Is More Fun Than Anywhere Else in Europe," *Culture Trip* (Updated Nov. 13, 2017), https://theculturetrip.com/europe/bosnia-herzegovina/articles/11-reasons-why-drinking-in-bosnia-is-more-fun-than-anywhere-else-in-europe/

40. Ritchie & Roser, note 39 ("Heavy Drinking Sessions").
41. "Bosnia And Herzegovina—Total Alcohol Consumption Per Capita," *Trading Econ.*, https://tradingeconomics.com/bosnia-and-herzegovina/total-alcohol-consumption-per-capita-liters-of-pure-alcohol-projected-estimates-15-years-of-age-wb-data.html
42. Ritchie & Roser, note 39.
43. Ibid.
44. Ibid.
45. Ibid.
46. Ante Ivanković et al., "Health Status of Population in Bosnia and Herzegovina in 15 Years of Transitional Period," *Antropol.* 34 (2010), Supp. 1: 331; Ritchie & Roser, note 39.
47. See "Bosnia and Herzegovina: Alcohol and Drug Use Disorders as a Share of Total Disease Burden, 1990 to 2016," *Our World in Data*, https://ourworldindata.org/grapher/alcohol-drug-use-disorders-share-total-dise ase?tab=chart&country=BIH (calculating the number for 2016 as 1.8%).
48. See Ritchie & Roser, note 39 ("The Health Impact of Alcohol").
49. "Smoking: An Endemic Problem in Bosnia and Herzegovina," *World Bank* (Nov. 20, 2012), http://www.worldbank.org/en/news/feature/2012/11/20/smoking-an-endemic-problem-in-bosnia-and-herzegovina, *archived at* https://perma.cc/H4YJ-H9U6 [hereinafter "Smoking in BiH"] (feature story on the International Tobacco Control Conference held in Sarajevo on November 5 and 6, 2012). See also Saša Petković et al., Accelerating Progress on Effective Tobacco Tax Policies in Low- and Middle-Income Countries: National Study—Bosnia and Herzegovina (University of Banja Luka, Bosnia and Herzegovina, 2018), pp. 5, 28, https://tobacconomics.org/wp-content/uploads/2019/02/National-study-BiH.pdf
50. See Smoking in BiH, note 49. In 2002, BiH boasted 37% of adult smokers, 49% of whom were men and 30% women. Two percent of pupils aged eleven to thirteen smoked cigarettes, while among the thirteen- to fifteen-year age bracket, 14% smoked, 17% of them boys and 10% girls. Ivanković et al., note 46, p. 331. See also Edin Jusufovic, "Hot Topics of Tobacco Control in Bosnia and Herzegovina," *Tobacco Prev. Cessation*, 4 (Supplement) (2018), A104, https://doi.org/10.18332/tpc/91065 (putting the prevalence rate at 26.7% for youth in the thirteen- to fifteen-year age bracket without breaking down the numbers into gender).
51. See "Share of People Who Smoke Every Day, 1980 to 2012," *Our World in Data*, https://ourworldindata.org/grapher/daily-smoking-prevalence?country=BIH (calculating the number as 31.2%).
52. "Bosnia and Herzegovina: Prevalence of Daily Smoking in Populations Aged 10 and Older, 1990 to 2016," *Our World in Data*, ourworldindata.org/grapher/prevalence-of-daily-smoking-sdgs?country=BIH

53. "Bosnia and Herzegovina: Prevalence of Tobacco Use among Adults, 2000 to 2016," *Our World in Data*, ourworldindata.org/grapher/prevalence-of-tobacco-use-sdgs?tab=chart&country=BIH
54. Ivanković et al., note 46, pp. 330–31.
55. Ibid., p. 331.
56. Smoking in BiH, note 49.
57. "Bosnia and Herzegovina: Death Rate from Smoking, 1990 to 2017," *Our World in Data*, https://ourworldindata.org/grapher/death-rate-smoking?country=BIH
58. Smoking in BiH, note 49.
59. See, for example, Carol Strong et al., "Effects of Adolescent Cigarette Smoking on Adulthood Substance Use and Abuse: The Mediating Role of Educational Attainment," *Subst. Use & Misuse*, 51(2) (2016), 141–54, doi: 10-3109/10826084.2015.1073323 (however finding no support in their data for the gateway hypothesis due perhaps to the mediating influence of educational attainment).
60. Smoking in BiH, note 49.
61. Ibid.
62. Ibid.
63. Ibid.
64. Ibid.
65. See, for example, World Health Org., *Regional Office for Eur., Tobacco Control Fact Sheet: Bosnia and Herzegovina* 1 (2016) [hereinafter *Tobacco Control Fact Sheet*] ("Based on the current level of adult smoking in Bosnia and Herzegovina [. . .] premature deaths attributable to smoking are projected to be as high as 600,000 of the more than 1.2 million smokers alive today [. . .] and may increase in the absence of stronger policies."). This fact sheet listed the following tobacco control policies, both for FBiH and RS (encapsulated in Tables 2 and, 3 respectively): smoke-free laws; services to help smokers quit; mass media anti-smoking campaigns; warnings on cigarette packages about the dangers of smoking; enforcing bans on tobacco advertising, promotion, and sponsorship; and raising taxes on tobacco products. Ibid., pp. 2–3. The report card on the war against tobacco in BiH, to the extent that such war exists, highlights the issue that indoor public places in BiH (such as healthcare facilities, educational facilities, government facilities, indoor offices and workplaces, restaurants, cafes, pubs and bars, and public transport) are not completely smoke-free. Ibid., p. 3 and tbl. 4. Similarly, bans on direct and indirect advertising in both FBiH and RS are still incomplete. See id., pp. 4–5 and tbls. 5–6.
66. Compare Smoking in BiH, note 49, with Tobacco Control Fact Sheet, note 65.

67. Jusufovic, note 50. See also Petković et al., note 49, pp. 19–23 (enumerating achievements in terms of legislation at the state and two entity levels).
68. Jusufovic, note 50.
69. See Huma Qureshi, "Smoking Shisha: How Bad Is It for You?" *Guardian* (London), (22 Aug. 2011), https://www.theguardian.com/society/2011/aug/22/shisha-smoking-how-bad-is-it
70. See ibid. Hookah is a smoking experience involving "a glass-bottomed water pipe in […] fruit-flavored tobacco […] covered with foil and roasted with charcoal." Ibid. The way hookah operates is that "[t]he tobacco smoke passes through a water chamber and is inhaled deeply and slowly; the fruit-flavored tobacco tastes smooth and smells sweet, enthusiasts say, making it an enjoyable and unrushed experience."
71. See ibid.
72. See ibid. But it feels like smoking, it needs to get the regulatory attention devoted to smoking products. This should probably get the attention electronic cigarettes (e-cigarettes) receive in the United States. E-cigarettes are classified as tobacco products, and manufacturers of these cigarettes indicate that they target smokers, not people seeking to quit. It is against this background that, in April 2014, the United States' Food and Drug Administration (FDA) proposed new regulations for tobacco products that include e-cigarettes. The regulations require disclosure of ingredients used in e-cigarette liquids, proof of safety of those ingredients, and regulation of the devices used to vaporize and deliver the liquid. In the United States, the FDA is responsible for protecting the public health by ensuring the safety, efficacy, and security of human and veterinary drugs, biological products, and medical devices; and by ensuring the safety of the country's food supply, cosmetics, and products that emit radiation.
73. See United Nations High Comm'r for Refugees' Office of the Chief of Mission in Bosnia. *Health Care in Bosnia and Herzegovina in the Context of the Return of Refugees and Displaced Persons* (Sarajevo: July), 18, 18 n.102    https://www.unhcr.org/news/updates/2001/7/3c614f6a4/health-care-bosnia-herzegovina-context-return-refugees-displaced-persons.html
74. Information is still sketchy, but by some recent estimates the state-level government contributed a minuscule 0.02% share to total expenditure on healthcare. Marko Martić & Ognjen Đukić, Friedrich Ebert Stiftung Sarajevo, "Health Care Systems in BiH: Financing Challenges and Reform Options?" (October 2017), 18 tbl. 5, https://library.fes.de/pdf-files/bueros/sarajevo/14124.pdf

75. "Bosnia and Herzegovina: Central Government Expenditure as Share of GDP, 2005 to 2016," *Our World in Data*, https://ourworldindata.org/grapher/total-gov-expenditure-gdp-wdi?tab=chart&country=BIH (calculating the number as 35.33%).

76. For a discussion on how wars negatively socialize individuals to pick up habits like smoking, which impact public health, see Associated Press, *Smoking in the Military: An Old Habit Dies Hard*, NBC News, http://www.nbcnews.com/id/32608436/ns/us_news-military/t/smoking-military-old-habit-dies-hard/#.XXpHESgzZPY, *archived at* https://perma.cc/323V-FLVX (focusing on the United States).

CHAPTER 8

# Conclusions

**Abstract** This chapter concludes the study with summational comments, including reflections on the theoretical contributions of the book to Bioethics, comparative healthcare studies, and comparative human right studies.

**Keywords** Preventive healthcare • The Affordable Care Act (ACA) in the United States • Bioethics • Comparative healthcare studies • Comparative human right studies

PREVENTIVE MEDICINE AS THE WAY FORWARD IN BOSNIA

This book is a contribution to the debate on healthcare reforms in postwar Bosnia built on the theory of preventive medicine, in turn anchored on genetic counseling, supplemented by the two public issues of alcohol and tobacco controls. Major highlights of the book are the four hallmarks it elaborated as a guide to healthcare reforms in Bosnia and the strategies for promoting preventive medicine through genetic counseling highlighted in the book. All of these themes are sensitive to healthcare as human right, consistent with a commitment to socioeconomic human rights, sincerely held yet not deep-rooted, that dates back to socialist Yugoslavia and is a carryover from that era.

Appropriately, this book ends as it began, with the Reform Agenda for Bosnia and Herzegovina 2015–2018.[1] Since 2015, with the support and encouragement of the international community,[2] Bosnia has unveiled

© The Author(s) 2020                                                    107
P. C. Aka, *Genetic Counseling and Preventive Medicine in Post-War Bosnia*, https://doi.org/10.1007/978-981-15-7987-5_8

reforms, healthcare included, designed to facilitate its integration into the European Union.[3] To be sure, on the surface, Bosnia's human development statistics looks generally good. This is evident in life expectancy, where the country ranks above average.[4] By the same token, compared to many countries in Europe, Bosnia exhibits low numbers,[5] bound to be improved through preventive medicine, via genetic counseling, backed by progress in alcohol and tobacco controls. As Bosnians strive to rebuild their economy after the devastations of an ethnic war that damaged their healthcare system, preventive healthcare in the expansive sense this book defined the term is the viable way forward.

Because today diseases morph from infectious to chronic categories,[6] prevention has assumed increased importance in healthcare administration and delivery. Thus, in the United States, the Affordable Care Act (ACA) under then president Barack Obama was predicated largely on preventive medicine.[7] This morphing of diseases into chronic categories also helps explain why, obviously from a preventive standpoint, newborns in the United States are screened for a panel of treatable genetic disorders.[8]

## REFLECTIONS ON THE THEORETICAL CONTRIBUTIONS OF THIS BOOK

Chapter 1 commented on the interdisciplinary character of this book, revolved around its setting in Bioethics, complemented and cemented by comparative healthcare studies, and comparative human right studies. The ensuing discussion reflects on the contributions of this book focused on healthcare reforms in Bosnia into these field. The goal is a statement more extensive than the comments provided in Chap. 1.

Bioethics is the application of ethics to medicine and healthcare.[9] The field focuses on the moral integrity of a community.[10] Bioethics takes its significance from its multidisciplinary character and insights, "bear[ing] on the complex interaction of human life, science, and technology."[11] Using philosophy and theology as point of departure, bioethicists draw and synthesize perspectives from various other disciplines, including medicine and other healthcare disciplines, sociology, anthropology, and law, which they in turn use to address issues of global healthcare, such as the purposes and ends of healthcare and the life sciences, and the meanings and implications of distributive justice, among other weighty issues.[12]

At the point of its birth in 1971, Bioethics "signified merely the combination of biology and bioscience with humanistic knowledge."[13] From this modest beginning, today the field has evolved to "encompass[ ] a full range of concerns, from difficult private decisions made in clinical settings, to controversies surrounding stem cell research, to implications of reproductive technologies, to broader concerns[,] such as international human subject research, to public policy in healthcare, and to the allocation of scarce resources."[14] Its application in this study, to which field this work on Bosnia equally contributes, speaks to the full spectrum.

Comparative analysis "entails "studying and comparing which solutions [...] work best for certain types of problems, as well as observing patterns of failure across multiple systems."[15] Healthcare is a primary political, economic, and social issue in many countries across the world, as well as a major focus of international concern.[16] Accordingly, as a field, comparative healthcare studies fosters full understanding of the dynamics of healthcare systems,[17] including cross-country learning and cooperation capable of generating evidence-based information that will help policymakers to rationalize the structure and funding of their healthcare systems.[18]

As the English writer Rudyard Kipling (1865–1936) once famously observed, he who knows only England knows not England well.[19] By the same token, studying other people's healthcare arrangements and experiences afford the examiner "multiple vantage points from which to gain a fresh perspective on strengths and weaknesses" of one's own healthcare system.[20] Comparison is also mandated by the fact that systems borrow from each other. For example, during the 1990s, Sweden adopted some of the healthcare reforms in the United Kingdom involving reorganization of primary care practices and shifting physician payment from fixed salary to capitation.[21]

Comparing healthcare systems can be daunting. It "entails a vast array of information, including historical background, cultural patterns and belief, geographic considerations, as well as an understanding of conceptual frameworks, theory, and comparative methods."[22] But "[t]he potential rewards of comparative work [...] balances the challenges."[23] Because many of the problems nations confront in delivering quality healthcare to their citizens are similar, "[t]here are lessons to be learned from comparing health-care systems internationally that can only aid in addressing these problems."[24]

Going beyond one nation state, familiarizing oneself with the what is good and bad with other people's healthcare reforms "provides a global laboratory for health systems development."[25] Cross-national, comparative research has the capacity to inform national policy debates within countries and across the world.[26] Heightened interest in comparative healthcare studies—the health reform experiences of other countries—coincided with the national debates in the United States on healthcare in the early 1990s under William J. Clinton.[27] Via this case study on Bosnia, this book adds to the heightened interests, at the same time comparative healthcare studies provide invaluable conceptual insights and themes that enriched this study.[28]

This occurrence calls to mind the advice of Karl Marx (1818–1883). In his Eleven Theses on Feuerbach, Marx advised his fellow philosophers to go beyond interpreting the world to actually changing it.[29] The same theme of interpretation as a springboard to action pervades the emerging field of comparative human rights. It is noticeable in the call for the adoption of a preventive approach to human rights by United Nations Secretary-General Ban Ki-moon.[30] It is also noticeable in the appeal by Samantha Power and her colleagues for scholars and policymakers to move from inspiration to impact in the attempt to realize human rights in a world where human right atrocities still galore, despite a flurry of domestic and international activities aimed at protecting and promoting these rights.[31] This work focused on Bosnia heeds the appeal to realize human rights, including its analysis of the healthcare debate in Bosnia anchored in preventive medicine from a human right standpoint.

## NOTES

1. See Chap. 1.
2. From 1996 to 2018, the United States provided assistance to Bosnia, in monetary terms, worth approximately US$2 billion. The assistance is in the areas of rebuilding infrastructure damaged during the Bosnian war, like health clinics, roads, bridges, power plants, power lines, water systems, and schools; creating jobs; reducing poverty in the rural areas; improving the Bosnian business environment; improving the efficiency of the justice system; promoting increased accountability and transparency; promoting tolerance and acceptance; and supporting marginalized and vulnerable groups, including children with disabilities. See "Fact Sheet: USAID Assistance in Bosnia and Herzegovina (1996-Present) (last updated May 22, 2018), https://www.usaid.gov/bosnia/fact-sheets/usaid-assistance-bosnia-and-herzegovina

3. See, for example, Reform Agenda for Bosnia and Herzegovina 2015–2018 (Working Translation) [hereinafter Reform Agenda for BiH], http://europa.ba/wp-content/uploads/2015/09/Reform-Agenda-BiH.pdf. (accessed July 22, 2019), ¶ 3 ("The priorities for reform were previously discussed with International Financial Institutions (IFIs) and the EU."); ibid. ¶ 2 ("All levels of government are mindful that meaningful progress on the implementation of the agenda for reform will be necessary for a membership application to be considered by the EU.").

4. See, for example, H. Plecher, "Bosnia and Herzegovina - Statistics and Facts," *Statista* (Feb. 8, 2019), https://www.statista.com/topics/4644/bosnia-and-herzegovina/, archived at https://perma.cc/NGS4-Z5FZ. For example, as this source points out, compared to other countries in Europe, life expectancy at birth in BiH is high. Ibid. In 2017, that number was 77.13 years. H. Plecher, "Life Expectancy at Birth in Bosnia & Herzegovina in 2017," *Statista* (Dec. 11, 2019), https://www.statista.com/statistics/452587/life-expectancy-at-birth-in-bosnia-herzegovina/, archived at https://perma.cc/PZ5T-S86B. See also United Nations Development Program, *Human Development Report 2019: Beyond Income, Beyond Averages, Beyond Today: Inequalities in Human Development in the twenty-first Century* (New York: United Nations Development Program, 2019) (showing that Bosnia was classified in the "high human development," a category over and above the two lower categories of "medium human development" and "low human development.")

5. See, for example, "Life Expectancy at Birth, Total (Years)," World Bank, https://data.worldbank.org/indicator/SP.DYN.LE00.IN, archived at https://perma.cc/9J9R-4SX8 (covering the period 1960–2017) (showing BiH has a life expectancy of seventy-seven, whereas it is eighty-three for Norway, France, and Italy, eighty-one for Germany and Slovenia, and seventy-eight for Albania). See also *Human Development Report 2019*, note 4 (showing countries like Turkey, Montenegro, Croatia, and Slovenia above Bosnia in the "very high human development" category).

6. See generally Siobhán M. O'Connor et al., "Emerging Infectious Determinants of Chronic Diseases," *Emerging Infectious Diseases*, 12(7) (2006), 1051 (2006); Inst. of Med., The Infectious Etiology of Chronic Diseases: Defining the Relationship, Enhancing the Research, and Mitigating the Benefits—Workshop Summary (Stacey L. Knobler et al. eds., National Academies Press 2004).

7. Patient Protection and Affordable Care Act, H.R. 3590, 111th Cong. (2010) (amended by Health Care and Education Reconciliation Act of 2010, Pub. L. No. 111–152, tit. IV, 124 Stat. 1029). See also "Preventive Services Covered Under the Affordable Care Act," Nat'l Conference of State Legislatures (February 2014), http://www.ncsl.org/research/

health/american-health-benefit-exchanges-b.aspx, *archived at* https://
perma.cc/B5GQ-TEFR; Vera Gruessner, "How the Affordable Care Act
Changed the Face of Health Insurance," *HealthPayer Intelligence* (June
15,   2016),   https://healthpayerintelligence.com/features/how-the-
affordable-care-act-changed-the-face-of-health-insurance, *archived at*
https://perma.cc/7GWF-NQK3 (discussing how the Act's "[p]reventive
medicine provisions incentivize accountable care"); Nadia Chait & Sherry
Glied, "Promoting Prevention Under the Affordable Care Act," *Ann. Rev.
Pub. Health*, 39 (2018), 507 (addressing the act's goals and specific
provisions).

8.  See Genetic Alliance, D.C. Dep't of Health, *Understanding Genetics: A
District of Columbia Guide for Patients and Health Professionals* (2010), 20
("Each year, more than 95% of all children born in the United States (at
least 4 million babies) are tested for a panel of diseases that, when detected
and treated early, can lead to significant reduction in disease severity and
possibly even prevention of the disease."). As this document elaborated,
"[w]ithin 48 hours of a child's birth," healthcare workers obtain samples,
called a 'blood spot,' from newborns. Then, they submit the blood for
testing at state-owned or state-approved laboratories, where it is "analyzed
for up to 50 diseases, including phenylketonuria (PKU), sickle cell disease,
and hypothyroidism." Ibid.

9.  "What is Bioethics," Center for Practical Ethics, https://practicalbioeth-
ics.org/what-is-bioethics

10. Ibid.

11. Ibid.

12. Ibid.

13. Ibid.

14. Ibid.

15. Mary Ko Zimmerman, "Comparative Health-Care Systems," *Encyclopedia
of Sociology* (updated Feb. 10, 2020), https://www.encyclopedia.com/
social-sciences/encyclopedias-almanacs-transcripts-and-maps/compara-
tive-health-care-systems ("Key Characteristics for the Comparison of
Health-Care Systems").

16. Marie L. Lassey et al., *Health Care Systems Around the World: Characteristics,
Issues, Reforms* (New York: Pearson, 1996) (book's back cover).

17. Zimmerman, note 15.

18. See Zsuzsanna Jakab, "Foreword from WHO," in Irene Papanicolas &
Peter C. Smith, eds., *Health System Performance Comparison: An Agenda
for Policy, Information[,] and Research* (Maidenhead, UK: Open University
Press, 2013), n.p.; and Irene Panniculus & Peter C. Smith, "Health
International Comparisons of Health Systems, *in* Papanicolas & Smith,
eds., *Health System Performance Comparison*, p. 75.

19. Rudyard Kipling, "The English Flag," *Bartleby.com* (1891), bartleby. com/364/122.html ("And what should they know of England who only England know?").
20. Zimmerman, note 15.
21. Ibid. ("Review of Selected Health-Care Systems"). Capitation payments "are fixed, pre-arranged monthly payments received by a physician, clinic or hospital per patient enrolled in a health plan, or per capita." Julia Kagan, "Capitation Payments," *Investopedia* (updated October 2, 2019), https://www.investopedia.com/terms/c/capitation-payments.asp. These payments are products of a capitated contract between a health insurance company and a healthcare provider. Ibid. In this contract, "[t]he monthly payment is calculated one year in advance and remains fixed for that year, regardless of how often the patient needs services." Ibid.
22. Zimmerman, note 15 ("Review of Selected Health-Care Systems").
23. Ibid. ("Review of Selected Health-Care Systems").
24. Ibid ("Review of Selected Health-Care Systems").
25. Ibid.
26. See Theodore R. Marmor, *Comparative Studies and the Politics of Modern Medical Care* (New Haven, CT: Yale Univ. Press, 2009) (essays covering policy debates and reforms in Canada, Germany, Holland, the United Kingdom, and the United States).
27. See ibid.
28. See Chap. 4. Comparative healthcare studies provided some of the gristmill for the guide to healthcare reforms in Bosnia embedded in human rights that the chapter proposed.
29. See Jonathan Wolff, "Karl Marx," *Stanford Encyclopedia of Philosophy* (Aug. 26, 2013, revised April 12, 2017), https://plato.stanford.edu/entries/marx/. Marx's Eleven Theses on Feuerbach is a short, iterative list concerning the work of Lugwig Feuerbach (1804–1872), a German philosopher and anthropologist known for his work critiquing Christianity. Feuerbach was a contemporary to Marx whose idea of alienation and religion heavily influenced Marx's views on alienation in society.
30. Rebecca M.M. Wallace & Olga Martin-Ortega, *International Law*, Seventh Ed. (London: Sweet & Maxwell, 2013), 319.
31. See generally Samantha Power & Graham Allison, eds., *Realizing Human Rights: Moving from Inspiration to Impact* (New York: St. Martin's Press, 2000).

# REFERENCES

*About Genetic Counselors: Genetic Counseling Prospective Student Frequently Asked Questions.* National Society of Genetic Counselors. https://www.nsgc.org/page/frequently-asked-questions-students, archived at https://perma.cc/KN2E-32Q2

Achebe, Chinua. 1964. *Arrow of God.* New York: Heinemann.

Additional Protocol to the Convention on Human Rights and Biomedicine on the Prohibition of Cloning Human Beings. 2007, January 9. C.E.T.S. No. 195.

Ahmetasevic, Nidzara. 2020. Bosnia and Herzegovina's COVID-19 Response Threatens Fragile Human Rights. *K2.0,* February 4. https://kosovotwopointzero.com/en/bosnia-and-herzegovinas-covid-19-response-threatens-fragile-human-rights/, archived at https://perma.cc/Q8Z5-4UXG

Aka, Philip C. 2006. Analyzing U.S. Commitment to Socioeconomic Human Rights. *Akron Law Review* 39: 417–463.

———. 2019. Fidel Castro and Socioeconomic Human Rights in Africa: A Multi-Level Analysis. *Fordham International Law Journal* 43 (Fall): 41–78.

Aka, Philip C., and Sencer Yeralan. 2019. Humor as Pedagogy: Evidence from Bosnia and Herzegovina. *Indonesian Journal of International & Comparative Law* VI (4): 539–603.

Aka, Philip C., et al. 2017. Ghana's National Health Insurance Scheme (NHIS) and the Evolution of a Human Right to Healthcare in Africa. *Chicago-Kent | Journal of International and Comparative Law* 17 (2): 1–65.

Allcock, John B., et al. n.d. *Balkans.* Encyclopedia Britannica. https://www.britannica.com/place/Balkans, archived at https://perma.cc/NG3U-JPAZ

American Society of Hematology. Frequently Asked Questions Regarding Sickle
Cell Trait. https://www.hematology.org/advocacy/policy-statements/2012/
faq-regarding-sickle-cell-trait, archived at https://perma.cc/9BFX-HQ5U
*An Introduction to the Public Policy-Making Cycle.* 2017. Point Park University
Online. June 14. https://online.pointpark.edu/public-administration/policy-
making-cycle/, available at https://perma.cc/ZF4E-G9L
ARUP Laboratories. 2016. *Cystic Fibrosis Carrier Testing: What You Need to
Know.* July. https://www.aruplab.com/files/resources/branding/Brochure_
patient_cystic.pdf
Associated Press. Smoking in the Military: An Old Habit Dies Hard. *NBC News,*
http://www.nbcnews.com/id/32608436/ns/us_news-military/t/smoking-
military-old-habit-dies-hard/#.XXpHESgzZPY, archived at https://perma.
cc/323V-FLVX
Ballantyne, Angela, et al. 2006. Medical Genetic Services in Developing Countries:
The Ethical, Legal and Social Implications of Genetic Testing and Screening.
https://apps.who.int/iris/bitstream/handle/10665/43288/924159344X_
eng.pdf?sequence=1&isAllowed=y
BAM—Bosnian Convertible Mark. *XE.* https://www.xe.com/currency/bam-
bosnian-convertible-mark, archived at https://perma.cc/8BLB-6N9Z
Baquet, James. 2010. A Stitch in Time Saves Nine. *Shenzhen Daily,* November 11.
http://www.szdaily.com/content/2010-11/11/content_5073819.htm,
archived at https://perma.cc/Z9WZ-C5J6
Bečar, Lejla. 2015. Alcoholism: The Socially Acceptable Disease. *Balkan Diskurs,*
July 26. https://balkandiskurs.com/en/2015/26/alcoholism-the-socially-
acceptable-disease/
Bedford, Sam. 2017. [Eleven] Reasons Why Drinking in Bosnia Is More Fun
Than Anywhere Else in Europe. *Culture Trip,* Updated Nov 13. https://the-
culturetrip.com/europe/bosnia-herzegovina/articles/11-reasons-why-
drinking-in-bosnia-is-more-fun-than-anywhere-else-in-europe/
Beganović, Šejma, et al. 2015. Huntington's Disease-Case Report. http://gyrus.
hiim.hr/images/suplement2/neuro2015_Part24.pdf
Ben-Senior, Liat. 2018. 10 Most Common Genetic Diseases. *LabRoots,* May 22.
labroots.com/trending/infographics/8833/10-common-genetic-diseases,
archived at https://perma.cc/H985-VX4L
BHMissionUN. https://bhmissionun.org/bosnia-and-herzegovina-un-3/,
archived at https://perma.cc/4TD4-4PX3
Bichta, Tomasz, ed. 2018. *Political Systems of the Former Yugoslavia: Bosnia and
Herzegovina, Croatia, Kosovo, Macedonia, Montenegro, Servia, and Slovenia.*
New York: Peter Lang.
*Bismarck versus Beveridge: A Comparison of Social Insurance Systems in Europe.*
2008. Cesifo Dice Report. April. https://www.ifo.de/DocDL/dicere-
port408-db6.pdf

Blatter, Werner. 2001. Foreword and Acknowledgments. In United Nations High Comm'r for Refugees' Office of the Chief of Mission in Bosnia. *Health Care in Bosnia and Herzegovina in the Context of the Return of Refugees and Displaced Persons*. Sarajevo, July. https://www.unhcr.org/news/updates/2001/7/3c614f6a4/health-care-bosnia-herzegovina-context-return-refugees-displaced-persons.html

Bojicic-Dzelilovic, Vesna. 2015. The Politics, Practice[,] and Paradox of 'Ethnic Security' in Bosnia-Herzegovina. *Stability: International Journal of Security and Development* 4 (1) art. 11.

Borry, Pascal, Mahsa Shabani, and Heidi Carmen Howard. 2014. Symposium: Is There a Right Time to Know? The Right Not to Know and Genetic Testing in Children. *Journal of Law Medicine and Ethics* 42 (1) 19, 20.

Borry, Pascal, et al. 2010. Where Are You Going, Where Have You Been: A Recent History of the Direct-to-Consumer Genetic Testing Market. *Journal of Community Genetics* 1 (3): 101.

Bosnia and Herzegovina. 2019. *Worldometer*, April 27. http://www.worldometers.info/world-population/bosnia-and-herzegovina-population/, archived at https://perma.cc/CJH7-3C7

Bosnia and Herzegovina GDP 1994-2018. *Trading Economics*. https://tradingeconomics.com/bosnia-and-herzegovina/gdp, archived at https://perma.cc/Y6DD-H3W

Bosnia and Herzegovina GDP Per Capita 1994-2018. *Trading Economics*. https://tradingeconomics.com/bosnia-and-herzegovina/gdp-per-capita, archived at https://perma.cc/Q8CF-PY45

*Bosnia and Herzegovina & UN*. Bosnia and Herzegovina Mission to the United Nations.

Bosnia and Herzegovina. Third Report of BiH on Implementation of the European Social Charter [Revised]. 2012, November. http://www.mhrr.gov.ba/PDF/LjudskaPrava/III%20IZVJESTAJ%20GRUPA%202%2%20eng.pdf

Bosnia and Herzegovina: Absolute Number of Deaths from Ambient Particulate Air Pollution, 1990 to 2015. *Our World in Data*. https://ourworldindata.org/grapher/absolute-number-of-deaths-from-ambient-particulate-air-pollution?tab=chart&country=BIH

Bosnia and Herzegovina: Alcohol and Drug Use Disorders as a Share of Total Disease Burden, 1990 to 2016. *Our World in Data*. https://ourworldindata.org/grapher/alcohol-drug-use-disorders-share-total-disease?tab=chart&country=BIH

Bosnia and Herzegovina: Central Government Expenditure as Share of GDP, 2005 to 2016. *Our World in Data*. https://ourworldindata.org/grapher/total-gov-expenditure-gdp-wdi?tab=chart&country=BIH

Bosnia and Herzegovina: Death Rate from Air Pollution (Per 100,000), 1990 to 2015. *Our World in Data.* https://ourworldindata.org/grapher/death-rate-from-air-pollution-per-100000?country=BIH

Bosnia and Herzegovina: Death Rate from Smoking, 1990 to 2017. *Our World in Data.* https://ourworldindata.org/grapher/death-rate-smoking?country=BIH

Bosnia and Herzegovina: Healthcare Access and Quality Index, 1990 to 2015. *Our World in Data.* https://ourworldindata.org/grapher/healthcare-access-and-quality-index?tab=chart&country=BIH

Bosnia and Herzegovina: Location, Size, and Extent. *Nations Encyclopedia.* http://www.nationsencyclopedia.com/Europe/Bosnia-and-Herzegovina-LOCATION-SIZE-AND-EXTENT.html, archived at https://perma.cc/V5CH-FWXW

Bosnia and Herzegovina: Prevalence of Daily Smoking in Populations Aged 10 and Older, 1990 to 2016. *Our World in Data.* ourworldindata.org/grapher/prevalence-of-daily-smoking-sdgs?country=BIH.

Bosnia and Herzegovina: Human Rights Scores, 1992 to 2017. *Our World in Data.* https://ourworldindata.org/grapher/human-rights-scores?tab=chart&time=1992..2017&country=~BIH

Bosnia and Herzegovina: Prevalence of Tobacco Use Among Adults, 2000 to 2016. *Our World in Data.* ourworldindata.org/grapher/prevalence-of-tobacco-use- sdgs? tab=chart&country=BIH

Bosnia and Herzegovina—Total Alcohol Consumption Per Capita. *Trading Economics.* https://tradingeconomics.com/bosnia-and-herzegovina/total-alcohol-consumption-per-capita-liters-of-pure-alcohol-projected-estimates-15-years-of-age-wb-data.html

Bosnia-Herzegovina Has Lost a Fifth of Its Pre-War Population, Census Shows. 2016. *Guardian* (London), July 1. https://www.theguardian.com/world/2016/jul/01/bosnia-herzegovina-has-lost-a-fifth-of-its-pre-war-population-census-shows

Bosnia and Herzegovina: Human Rights Violations, 2006 to 2014. *Our World in Data.* https://ourworldindata.org/grapher/human-rights-violations?tab=chart&time=2006..2014&country=~BIH

Bowditch, Caroline. Genetic Counseling. *Encyclopedia Britannica.* https://www.britannica.com/science/genetic-counselling, archived at https://perma.cc/HR8G-KTSJ

Branković, Azra. 2016. Administrative Structure of Bosnia and Herzegovina. In *Bosnia and Herzegovina: Law, Society[,] and Politics,* ed. Yucel Oğurlu and Ahmed Mulanić, 10–30. Sarajevo: International University of Sarajevo.

Brothers, Kyle B., and Mark A. Rothstein. 2015. Ethical, Legal, and Social Implications of Incorporating Personalized Medicine into Healthcare. *Personalized Medicine* 12 (1): 43–51.

Brunner, Borga, and David Johnson. 2017. Timeline: Former Yugoslavia: From World War I to the Splintering of the Country. *Infoplease.* Updated Feb 28. https://www.infoplease.com/history/world/timeline-the-former-yugoslavia

Burci, Gian Luca, and Claude-Henri Vignes. 2004. *World Health Organization.* Zuidpoolsingel, Netherlands: Kluwer Law International.

Burg, Steven L., and Paul S. Shoup. 1999. *The War in Bosnia-Herzegovina: Ethnic Conflict and International Intervention.* 2nd ed. Armonk: M.E. Sharpe.

Cabrera, Oscar A., and Lawrence O. Gostin. 2013. Global Tobacco Control: A Vital Component of the Right to Health. In *Advancing the Human Right to Health,* ed. José M. Zuniga et al., 261–274. New York: Oxford University Press.

Cain, Jennifer, et al., eds. 2002. *Health Care Systems in Transition: Bosnia and Herzegovina.* Copenhagen: European Observatory on Health Care Systems.

Carballo, M., et al. 1997. Development of an Essential Drug List for Bosnia and Herzegovina. *Journal of the Royal Society of Medicine* 90 (June): 331–333. http://europepmc.org/backend/ptpmcrender.fcgi?accid=PMC1296311& blobtype=pdf

Catic, Tarik, and Selma Skrbo. 2013. Pharmacoeconomic Education for Pharmacy Students in Bosnia and Herzegovina. *Materia Socio Medica [Journal of Academy of Medical Sciences of Bosnia and Herzegovina]* 25 (4): 282–283.

Centers for Disease Control and Prevention. *What Is Hemophilia?* https://www. cdc.gov/ncbddd/hemophilia/facts.html, archived at https://perma. cc/XX7U-FYM5

Central Intelligence Agency. 2019. Bosnia and Herzegovina. *CIA World Factbook.* Updated Sept 24. https://www.cia.gov/library/publications/the-world-fact-book/geos/bk.html

———. "North Macedonia." *The World Factbook.* https://www.cia.gov/library/publications/the-world-factbook/geos/mk.html

Chait, Nadia, and Sherry Glied. 2018. Promoting Prevention Under the Affordable Care Act. *Annual Review of Public Health* 39: 507.

Chan, Margaret. 2010. Message from the Director-General. In *The World Health Report: Health Systems Financing: The Path to Universal Coverage,* ed. World Health Organization, vi–vii. Geneva: World Health Organization.

Chappelow, Jim. 2019. Pareto Efficiency. *Investopedia.* Updated Sept 25. https:// www.investopedia.com/terms/p/pareto-efficiency.asp

Chapter IV—Human Rights: 3. International Covenant on Economic, Social and Cultural Rights. United Nations Treaty Collection. https://treaties.un.org/ Pages/ViewDetails.aspx?src=IND&mtdsg_no=IV-3&chapter=4&lang=en, archived at https://perma.cc/N22X-CNM

Cherry, Kendra. The Age Old Debate of Nature vs. Nurture. *VeryWellMind.* https://www.verywellmind.com/what-is-nature-versus-nurture-2795392, archived at https://perma.cc/KQ6G-JBNQ

Chokoshvili, Davit, et al. 2017. Public Views on Genetics and Genetic Testing: A Survey of the General Public in Belgium. *Genetic Testing & Molecular Biomarkers* 21 (3): 195.

Clinton, Hilary Rodham. 2006. *It Takes a Village*, 10th Anniversary ed. New York: Simon & Schuster. (originally published in 1996).

Coggi, Paola Testori. 2013. Foreword from the European Commission. In *Health System Performance Comparison: An Agenda for Policy Information and Research*, ed. Irene Papanicolas and Peter C. Smith, xi–xii. Maidenhead: Open University Press.

Collins, R.E., et al. 2011. Impact of Communicating Personalized Genetic Risk Information on Perceived Control Over the Risk: A Systematic Review. *Genetics in Medicine: Official Journal of American College of Medical Genetics* 13 (4): 273–277.

Comparative Analysis: Definition, Concepts, and Writing Techniques. 2015. *Writeawriting*, April 14. https://www.writeawriting.com/academic-writing/comparative-analysis/

Constitution of Bosnia and Herzegovina. Annex 4 to the General Framework Agreement for Peace in Bosnia and Herzegovina. 1995. http://www.ohr.int/ohr-dept/legal/laws-of-bih/pdf/001%20-%20Constitutions/BH/BH%20CONSTITUTION%20.pdf

Constitution of Republika Srpska. 1992. Official Gazette of Republika Srpska No. 21/92 – consolidated version, 28/94, 8/96, 13/96, 15/96, 16/96, 21/96, 21/02, 26/02, 30/02, 31/02, 69/02, 31/03, 98/03, 115/05, 117/05, 48/11), available at http://www.ohr.int/ohr-dept/legal/laws-of-bih/pdf/001%20-%20Constitutions/RS/RS%20CONSTITUTION%20OF%20REPUBLIKA%20SRPSKA.pdf

Constitution of the Federation of Bosnia and Herzegovina. 1994. Official Gazette of the Federation of Bosnia and Herzegovina, 1/94. https://advokat-prnjavorac.com/legislation/constitution_fbih.pdf

Corley, Jacquelyn. 2020. U.S. Government Response to COVID-19 Was Slow. But How Does It Compare to Other Countries? *Forbes*, April 10. https://www.forbes.com/sites/jacquelyncorley/2020/04/10/us-government-response-to-covid-19-was-slow-but-how-does-it-compare-to-other-countries/, archived at https://perma.cc/EBH9-BTAW

Council of Europe. 1997. Convention for the Protection of Human Rights and Dignity of the Human Being with regard to the Application of Biology and Medicine: Convention on Human Rights and Biomedicine. ETS No. 164.

———. 2018. *Action Plan for Bosnia and Herzegovina 2018-2021*. (Jun. 13). https://rm.coe.int/bih-action-plan-2018-2021-en/16808b7563

———. 2019. *Bosnia and Herzegovina and the European Social Charter* [Factsheet]. rm.coe.int/pdf/1680492808, archived at https://perma.cc/YV7U-VEVL

Council of Europe, Committee of Ministers, Recommendation No. R (92) 3 on Genetic Testing and Screening for Health Care Purposes. 1992. (February 10). *Reprinted in Int'l Digest of Health Legislation*, 43: 284, http://hrlibrary.umn. edu/instree/coerecr92-3.html

Council of Europe. Parliamentary Assembly. 2018. *The Honoring of Obligations and Commitments by Bosnia and Herzegovina*. (Doc. No. 14465). (Jan. 8).

Countries. World Health Organization. https://www.who.int/countries/en/#B, archived at https://perma.cc/7C8L-QZ3T

Craig, Tara. 2014. Healthcare Marketing Compliance in the UK—Prevention Beats Cure. *PMLive*, July 1. https://www.pmlive.com/pharma_intelligence/healthcare_marketing_compliance_in_the_uk_-prevention_beats_cure_581532, archived at https://perma.cc/BPW7-EZ33

Crampton, Richard J. Balkans. *Encyclopedia Britannica*, https://www.britannica.com/place/Balkans

Croatia Population 2020. n.d. *World Population Review*. https://worldpopulationreview.com/countries/croatia-population/, archived at https://perma.cc/9LXA-F8RJ

Decision on the Base and Rate of Contribution for Health Insurance. Official Gazette of the Brčko District of BiH, 37/2009.

Donnelly, Jack. 2013. *Universal Human Rights in Theory and Practice*. 3rd ed. Ithaca: Cornell Univ. Press.

Dressler, Lynne G., et al. 2014. Genomics Education for the Public: Perspectives of Genomic Researchers and ELSI Advisors. *Genetic Testing & Molecular Biomarkers* 18 (3): 131, 138.

Drobes, David J. Nat'l Inst. on Alcohol Abuse and Alcoholism. 2002. *Concurrent Alcohol and Tobacco Dependence*. (Nov.). https://pubs.niaaa.nih.gov/publications/arh26-2/136-142.htm

Duchenne Muscular Dystrophy | Niche and Rare Pharmacor | G7 |. 2015. DRG (Dec.). https://decisionresourcesgroup.com/report/141434-biopharma-duchenne-muscular-dystrophy-niche-and-rare/, archived at https://perma.cc/SJP6-N58E

Duchenne UK. 2019. *Girls Living with Duchenne*. https://www.duchenneuk.org/girls-living-with-duchenne, archived at https://perma.cc/929Z-EFYN

The Eighth Global Conference on Health Promotion, Helsinki, Finland, 10–14 June 2013. The Helsinki Statement on Health in All Policies.

Epstein, Charles J. 2003. Is Modern Genetics the New Eugenics? *Genetics in Medicine* 5: 469–475. https://www.nature.com/gim/journal/v5/n6/full/gim2003376a.html.

Epstein, Lita. 2019. 6 Reasons Healthcare Is So Expensive in the U.S. *Investopedia*. Updated July 30. https://www.investopedia.com/articles/personal-finance/080615/6-reasons-healthcare-so-expensive-us.asp, archived at https://perma.cc/YD8V-6TPN

Europe: Bosnia and Herzegovina. n.d. *Center Intelligence Agency: The World Factbook.* https://www.cia.gov/library/publications/the-world-factbook/geos/bk.html, archived at https://perma.cc/3HMA-XXXX

European Social Charter (Revised). 1996. E.T.S. No. 163. rm.coe.int/168007cf93

Executive Summary: Why Universal Coverage? 2010. *The World Health Report: Health Systems Financing: The Path to Universal Coverage,* ix–xxii. Geneva: World Health Organization.

Fabinger, Jakov. 2020. Ethiopian Airlines Flies Huge Boeing 777 to Tiny Bosnian Town. *Simple Flying,* April 24. https://simpleflying.com/ethiopian-airlines-bosnian-town/, archived at https://perma.cc/47BZ-YMB4

Fact Sheet: USAID Assistance in Bosnia and Herzegovina (1996-Present). 2018. (Last updated May 22). https://www.usaid.gov/bosnia/fact-sheets/usaid-assistance-bosnia-and-herzegovina

Fahy, Nick. 2013. Commentary on International Health System Performance Information. In *Health System Performance Comparison: An Agenda for Policy, Information and Research,* ed. Irene Papanicolas and Peter C. Smith, 313–334. Maidenhead: Open University Press.

Farago, Jason. 2018. When Yugoslavia's Bright Future Was Fashioned in Concrete. *Wral,* July 19. https://www.wral.com/when-yugoslavia-s-bright-future-was-fashioned-in-concrete/17708739/

Florimon, Hector. 2019. Why the US Spends More on Health Care Than Other Countries, But Doesn't Fare Better: Study. *ABC News,* September 12. https://abcnews.go.com/Health/us-spends-health-care-countries-fare-study/story?id=53710650

Führer, Michaela. 2011. Bosnia-Herzegovina's Political System. *DW,* October 25. https://www.dw.com/en/bosnia-herzegovinas-political-system/a-15486583, archived at https://perma.cc/GT9X-ZMT

Gavrić, Saša, et al. 2013. *The Political System of Bosnia and Herzegovina: Institutions, Actors, Processes.* Sarajevo: Sarajevo Open Center.

The General Framework Agreement for Peace in Bosnia and Herzegovina. 1995. (Dec. 14). Yugoslavia–Bosn. & Herz.–Croatia. https://www.osce.org/bih/126173?download=true

Genetic Alliance. D.C. Dep't of Health. 2010. *Understanding Genetics: A District of Columbia Guide for Patients and Health Professionals.* Washington, DC: District of Columbia.

Genetic Counseling. *Merriam-Webster.* merriam-webster.com/dictionary/genetic%20counseling, archived at https://perma.cc/HJG6-8HQ2

Goldstein, Ellen, et al. 2015. Three Reasons Why the Economy of Bosnia and Herzegovina is Off Balance. *Brookings Future Development,* November 5. https://www.brookings.edu/blog/future-development/2015/11/05/three-reasons-why-the-economy-of-bosnia-and-herzegovina-is-off-balance

Gottesman, M.M., and F.S. Collins. 1994. Symposium: The Role of the Human Genome Project in Disease Prevention. *Preventive Medicine* 23 (5): 591–94.

Gruessner, Vera. 2016. How the Affordable Care Act Changed the Face of Health Insurance. *HealthPayer Intelligence*, June 15. https://healthpayerintelligence. com/features/how-the-affordable-care-act-changed-the-face-of-health-insurance, archived at https://perma.cc/7GWF-NQK3

Guzvic, Vladmiri, et al. 2018. Rare Diseases and Orphan Drugs Accessibility in Bosnia and Herzegovina. *Materia Socio Medica [Journal of Academy of Medical Sciences of Bosnia and Herzegovina]* 30 (4): 297–298.

Haga, Susanne B., et al. 2019. Primary Care Physicians' Knowledge, Attitudes, and Experience with Personal Genetic Testing. *Journal of Personalized Medicine* 9 (2): 29, 37–8.

Hauser, Diane, et al. 2018. Views of Primary Care Providers on Testing Patients for Genetic Risks for Common Chronic Diseases. *Health Affairs* 37 (5): 793, 794.

Healthcare in Bosnia-Herzegovina. *Best Country*, http://www.best-country. com/europe/bosnia_herzegovina/medicine

Heymann, David, and Robert Yates. 2014. *Embracing the Politics of Universal Health Coverage*. Chatham House: The Royal Institute of International Affairs. https://www.chathamhouse.org/expert/comment/embracing-politics-universal-health-coverage, archived at https://perma.cc/65KF-K5LV

History of the Human Genome Project. Human Genome Project Info. Archive 1990-2003. https://web.ornl.gov/sci/techresources/Human_Genome/project/hgp.shtml, archived at https://perma.cc/E5P8-EFEQ

Horowitz, Michael D., et al. 2007. Medical Tourism: Globalization of the Healthcare Marketplace. *Medscape General Medicine* 9 (4): 33.

Howard, Heidi C., and Pascal Borry. 2013. Survey of European Clinical Geneticists on Awareness, Experiences, and Attitudes toward Direct-to-Consumer Genetic Testing. *Genome Medicine* 5 (5): 45.

Huterer, Dražen, et al. 2013. Bosnian Divisions Create Bureaucratic Headaches. *Pro.Ba*. https://pro.ba/en/bosnia-divisions-create-bureaucratic-headaches/, archived at https://perma.cc/N2BH-MQ97

Institute of Medicine, Div. of Health Sci. Policy, Comm. On Assessing Genetic Risks. 1994. In *Assessing Genetic Risks: Implications for Health and Social Policy*, ed. Lori B. Andrews et al. Washington, DC: National Academies Press.

Institute of Medicine. Stacey L. Knobler, et al. 2004. *The Infectious Etiology of Chronic Diseases: Defining the Relationship, Enhancing the Research, and Mitigating the Effects—Workshop Summary*. Washington, DC: National Academies Press.

International Covenant on Economic, Social, and Cultural Rights. 1976. U.N. General Assembly Resolution No. 2200A (XXI) (19 December 1966), 993 U.N.T.S. 3.

Ivanković, Ante, et al. 2010. Health Status of Population in Federation of Bosnia and Herzegovina in 15 Years of Transitional Period. *Collegium Antropologicum* 34 (Supp. 1): 330–331.

Jakab, Zsuzsanna. 2013. Foreword from WHO. In *Health System Performance Comparison: An Agenda for Policy, Information and Research*, ed. Irene Papanicolas and Peter C. Smith. Maidenhead: Open University Press.

Javanović, Svetlana. 2018. Sarajevo World's Most Polluted City, Poor Air Quality Seen Across Western Balkans. *Balkan Green Energy News*, December 4. https://balkangreenenergynews.com/sarajevo-worlds-most-polluted-city-poor-air-quality-seen-across-western-balkans/

Jewell, Jennifer A. Fragile X Syndrome. *Medscape*. https://emedicine.medscape.com/article/943776-overview, archived at https://perma.cc/96AL-RZ78

Judah, Tim. 2019. Bosnia Powerless to Halt Demographic Decline. *BalkanInsight*, November 21. https://balkaninsight.com/2019/11/21/bosnia-powerless-to-halt-demographic-decline/

Jusufovic, Edin. 2018. Hot Topics of Tobacco Control in Bosnia and Herzegovina. *Tobacco Prevention and Cessation* 4 (Supplement): A104. https://doi.org/10.18332/tpc/91065.

Kagan, Julia. 2019. Capitation Payments. *Investopedia*. Updated Oct 2. https://www.investopedia.com/terms/c/capitation-payments.asp

Kalokairinou, Louiza, et al. 2018. Legislation of Direct-to-Consumer Genetic Testing in Europe: A Fragmentary Regulatory Landscape. *Journal of Community Genetics* 9 (2): 117–132.

Karanikolos, Marina, et al. 2013. Comparing Population Health. In *Health System Performance Comparison: An Agenda for Policy Information and Research*, ed. Irene Papanicolas and Peter C. Smith, 127–156. Maidenhead: Open University Press.

Keil, Soeren. 2012. Federalism as a Tool of Conflict-Resolution: The Case of Bosnia and Herzegovina. *Dans L'Europe en Formation [Europe in Formation]* 1 (363): 205. https://www.cairn.info/revue-l-europe-en-formation-2012-1-page-205.htm

Kenton, Will, and Brian Abbott. 2019. Moral Hazard. *Investopedia*. Updated Apr 10. https://www.investopedia.com/terms/m/moralhazard.asp, archived at https://perma.cc/Z9XK-NAKJ

Khan, Sarah A. 2019a. Bosnian Resurrection. *Arkansas Democrat Gazette*, July 7. https://www.arkansasonline.com/news/2019/jul/07/resurrection-20190707/

———. 2019b. Bosnia and Herzegovina: Still Fighting But This Time for Life. *Independent (UK)*, May 28. https://www.independent.co.uk/travel/bosnia-and-herzegovina-war-new-life-travel-visit-a8925981.html

Kingdom of Serbs, Croats, and Slovenes: Historical Kingdom, Balkans [1918–1929]. n.d. *Encyclopedia Britannica*. https://www.britannica.com/

place/Kingdom-of-Serbs-Croats-and-Slovenes, archived at https://perma. cc/BCL2-8HV6

Kipling, Rudyard. 1891. The English Flag. *Bartleby.com*. bartleby. com/364/122.html

Krulwich, Robert. 2003. Cracking the Code of Life. *PBS Television Show*. pbs.org. wgbh/nova/genome/

Kunitz, Stephen J. 2004. The Making and Breaking of Yugoslavia and Its Impact on Health. *American Journal of Public Health* 94 (11): 1894.

Kurtovic-Kozaric, Amina, et al. 2016. Ten-Year Trends in Prevalence of Down Syndrome in a Developing Country: Impact of the Maternal Age and Prenatal Screening. *European Journal of Obstetrics and Gynecology and Reproductive Biology* 206: 79. https://www.ejog.org/article/S0301-2115(16)30894-6/pdf

———. 2016. Diagnostics of Common Microdeletion Syndromes Using Fluorescence *in situ* Hybridization: Single Center Experience in a Developing Country. *Bosnian Journal of Basic Medical Sciences* 16 (2): 121. https://www. bjbms.org/ojs/index.php/bjbms/article/view/994/26

Lakic, Mladen. 2018. Bosnian Entrepreneurs Face Bureaucratic Obstacles to Success. *BalkanInsight*, November 7. https://balkaninsight. com/2018/11/07/bosnian-entrepreneurs-struggling-with-administration-amid-creative-ideas-11-06-2018/, archived at https://perma.cc/4T8Y-KDX

Lampe, John R. Bosnian War: European History [1992–1995]. *Encyclopedia Britannica*. https://www.britannica.com/event/Bosnian-War

Lampe, John R., and John B. Allcock. Yugoslavia: Former Federated Nation [1929-2003]. *Encyclopedia Britannica*. https://www.britannica.com/place/ Yugoslavia-former-federated-nation-1929-2003, archived at https://perma. cc/Q2FB-8TL4

Lassey, Marie L., et al. 1996. *Health Care Systems Around the World: Characteristics, Issues, Reforms*. New York: Pearson.

The Law on Health Care. Official Gazette of Republika Srpska, No. 18/99.

The Law on Health Care. Federation of Bosnia and Herzegovina. 2010 and 2013. Official Gazette of the Federation of Bosnia and Herzegovina, 46/10, and 75/13.

The Law on Health Insurance. Official Gazette of Republika Srpska, No. 18/99.

The Law on Health Insurance, Federation of Bosnia and Herzegovina. Official Gazette of the Federation of Bosnia and Herzegovina, 30/97, 7/02, 70/08, and 48/11.

Lee, Kelley. 2008. *Global Institutions: The World Health Organization (WHO)*. Abingdon: Routledge.

Legge, James. 1971. *Confucian Analects, The Great Learning, and the Doctrine of the Mean*. Mineola: Dover Publications.

Lewis, Ricki. 2014. Genetic Testing for All: Is It Eugenics? *DNA Science: Genetics in Context.* Posted September 18. http://blogs.plos.org/dnascience/2014/09/18/genetic-testing-eugenics/

Lobo, Ingrid. 2008. Environmental Influences on Gene Expression. *Nature Education* 1 (1): 39.

Lobo, Ingrid, and Kira Zhaurova. 2008. Birth Defects: Causes and Statistics. *Nature Education* 1 (1): 18. https://www.nature.com/scitable/topicpage/birth-defects-causes-and-statistics-863/

Lwoff, Laurence. 2009. Council of Europe Adopts Protocol on Genetic Testing for Health Purposes. *European Journal of Human Genetics* 17 (11): 1374–1377.

Mahmutovic, Lejla, et al. 2018. Perceptions of Students in Health and Molecular Life Sciences Regarding Pharmacogenomics and Personalized Medicine. *Human Genomics* 12 (1): 50.

Manolio, Teri A., et al. 2015. Global Implementation of Genomic Medicine: We Are Not Alone. *Science Translational Medicine* 7 (290), 290ps13. https://doi.org/10.1126/scitranslmed.aab0194.

Marmor, Theodore R. 2009. *Comparative Studies and the Politics of Modern Medical Care.* New Haven: Yale University Press.

Martić, Marko, and Ognjen Đukić. 2017. Friedrich Ebert Stiftung Sarajevo. *Health Care Systems in BiH: Financing Challenges and Reform Options?* October 20. https://library.fes.de/pdf-files/bueros/sarajevo/14124.pdf

Mayo Clinic. *Sickle Cell Anemia.* https://www.mayoclinic.org/diseases-conditions/sickle-cell-anemia/symptoms-causes/syc-20355876, archived at https://perma.cc/A3FJ-LHVE

———. *Thalassemia.* https://www.mayoclinic.org/diseases-conditions/thalassemia/symptoms-causes/syc-20354995, archived at https://perma.cc/4S2A-QMC4

McCuaig, Jeanna M., et al. 2018. Next Generation Service Delivery: A Scoping Review of Patient Outcomes Associated with Alternative Models of Genetic Counseling and Genetic Testing for Hereditary Cancer. *Cancers (Basel)* 10 (11): 435. https://doi.org/10.3390/cancers10110435.

McElheny, Victor K. 2010. *Drawing the Map of Life: Inside the Human Genome Project.* New York: Basic Books.

Medicine in Bosnia-Herzegovina. 2019. *Best Country*, August 27. http://www.best-country.com/europe/bosnia_herzegovina/medicine, archived at https://perma.cc/758U-J5D

Mikulic, Matej. 2019. Health Expenditure as a Percentage of Gross Domestic Product in Selected Countries in 2017. *Statista*, November 12. https://www.statista.com/statistics/268826/health-expenditure-as-gdp-percentage-in-oecd-countries/, archived at https://perma.cc/LXY7-AUFQ.

National Human Genome Research Institute. *Human Genome Project Completion: Frequently Asked Questions.* genome.gov/human_genome_project/Completion-FAQ

———. *FAQ.* https://www.genome.gov/human-genome-project/Completion-FAQ, archived at https://perma.cc/8BLR-VLDK

National Institute of Health, U.S. National Library of Medicine. *What Are Genome Editing and CRISPR-Cas9?* https://ghr.nlm.nih.gov/primer/genomicresearch/genomeediting

National Organization for Rare Disorders. 2016. *Rare Disease Database: Duchenne Muscular Dystrophy.* https://rarediseases.org/rare-diseases/duchenne-muscular-dystrophy/, archived at https://perma.cc/S38A-8U4W

———. 2017. *Rare Disease Database: Tay Sachs Disease.* https://rarediseases.org/rare-diseases/tay-sachs-disease/, archived at https://perma.cc/6334-28J

———. 2018. *Rare Disease Database: Angelman Syndrome.* https://rarediseases.org/rare-diseases/angelman-syndrome/, archived at https://perma.cc/RTB8-N7K3

Ndebele, Paul, and Rosemary Musesengwa. 2008. Will Developing Countries Benefit from Their Participation in Genetics Research? *Malawi Medical Journal* 20 (2): 67.

Noori, Tayebeh, et al. 2019. International Comparison of Thalassemia Registries: Challenges and Opportunities. *Acta Informatica Medica [Journal of Academy of Medical Sciences of Bosnia and Herzegovina]* 27 (1): 58. https://www.ncbi.nlm.nih.gov/pmc/articles/PMC6511274

Novo, Ahmed, et al. 2019. Measures to Improve Integration of Healthcare in Federation of Bosnia and Herzegovina. *Materia Socio Medica [Journal of Academy of Medical Sciences of Bosnia and Herzegovina]* 31 (1): 71.

O'Connor, Siobhán M., et al. 2006. Emerging Infectious Determinants of Chronic Diseases. *Emerging Infectious Diseases* 12 (7): 1051.

O'Donnell, Peter H., et al. 2017. Pharmacogenomics-Based Point-of-Care Clinical Decision Support Significantly Alters Drug Prescribing. *Clinical Pharmacology & Therapeutics* 102 (5): 859.

Office of High Representative. 2017. 51st Report of the High Representative for Implementation of the Peace Agreement on Bosnia and Herzegovina to the Secretary-General of the United Nations. (May 17). http://www.ohr.int/?p=97409

Paneque, Milena, et al. 2016. Development of a Registration System for Genetic Counsellors and Nurses in Health-care Services in Europe. *European Journal of Human Genetics* 24: 312.

Papanicolas, Irene, and Peter C. Smith. 2013. International Comparisons of Health Systems. In *Health System Performance Comparison: An Agenda for Policy Information and Research,* ed. Irene Papanicolas and Peter C. Smith, 75–112. Maidenhead: Open University Press.

Patient Protection and Affordable Care Act, H.R. 3590, 111th Cong. (2010) (amended by Health Care and Education Reconciliation Act of 2010, Pub. L. No. 111-152, tit. IV, 124 Stat. 1029).

Pawlson, I. Gregory, et al. 2019. Healthcare Systems. *Encyclopedia of Bioethics.* Updated Dec 4. https://www.encyclopedia.com/science/encyclopedias-almanacs-transcripts-and-maps/healthcare-systems

Peters, David H., et al. 2008. Poverty and Access to Health Care in Developing Countries. *Annals of the New York Academy of Sciences* 1136: 161–171. https://doi.org/10.1196/annals.1425.011.

Petković, Saša, et al. 2018. *Accelerating Progress on Effective Tobacco Tax Policies in Low- and Middle-Income Countries: National Study—Bosnia and Herzegovina.* Banja Luka, Bosnia and Herzegovina: University of Banja Luka. https://tobacconomics.org/wp-content/uploads/2019/02/National-study-BiH.pdf

Phillips, Kathryn A., et al. 2018. Genetic Test Availability and Spending: Where Are We Now? Where Are We Going? *Health Affairs* 37 (5): 710.

Plecher, H. 2019a. Bosnia and Herzegovina—Statistics and Facts. *Statista*, February 8. https://www.statista.com/topics/4644/bosnia-and-herzegovina/, archived at https://perma.cc/NGS4-Z5F

———. 2019b. Life Expectancy at Birth in Bosnia & Herzegovina in 2017. *Statista*, December 11. https://www.statista.com/statistics/452587/life-expectancy-at-birth-in-bosnia-herzegovina/, archived at https://perma.cc/PZ5T-S86B

Power, Samantha, and Graham Allison, eds. 2000. *Realizing Human Rights: Moving from Inspiration to Impact.* New York: St. Martin's Press.

*Preventive Services Covered Under the Affordable Care Act.* 2014. National Conference of State Legislatures, February. http://www.ncsl.org/research/health/american-health-benefit-exchanges-b.aspx, archived at https://perma.cc/B5GQ-TEFR

Qureshi, Huma. 2011. Smoking Shisha: How Bad Is It for You? *Guardian* (London), August 22. https://www.theguardian.com/society/2011/aug/22/shisha-smoking-how-bad-is-it

Rantanen, Elina. 2014. *Expectations, Frames[,] and Practices of Genetic Counselling in Different Contexts of Genetic Testing.* Ph.D. diss., University of Turku, Finland, 2014. https://www.utupub.fi/bitstream/handle/10024/98897/Annales%20D%20130%20Rantanen%20DISS.pdf?sequence=2&isAllowed=y

Rantanen, Elina, et al. 2006. Regulations and Practices Related to Genetic Counselling in 38 European Countries. www.eurogentest.org/fileadmin/templates/eugt/pdf/Results_of_survey_1_WP_3-1_Dec06.pdf

Rare Disease Database: Angelman Syndrome. National Organization for Rare Disorders. https://rarediseases.org/rare-diseases/angelman-syndrome/, archived at https://perma.cc/RTB8-N7K3

Rare Disease Database: Duchenne Muscular Dystrophy. National Organization for Rare Disorders. https://rarediseases.org/rare-diseases/duchenne-muscular-dystrophy/, archived at https://perma.cc/S38A-8U4W

Rare Disease Database: Tay Sachs Disease. National Organization for Rare Disorders. https://rarediseases.org/rare-diseases/tay-sachs-disease/, archived at https://perma.cc/6334-28JR

Reform Agenda for Bosnia and Herzegovina 2015-2018 (Working Translation). http://europa.ba/wp-content/uploads/2015/09/Reform-Agenda-BiH.pdf, archived at https://perma.cc/X385-JW5K

Remembering Generation that Rebuilt Our Country: Happy Statehood Day of BiH! 2019. *Sarajevo Times*, November 29. https://www.sarajevotimes.com/remembering-generation-that-rebuilt-our-country-happy-statehood-day-of-bih-2/

Ritchie, Hannah, and Max Roser. 2019 (2018). Alcohol Consumption. *Our World in Data*. April 2018, updated Nov 2019. https://ourworldindata.org/alcohol-consumption

Roberts, Marc J., et al. 2019 (paperback; originally published 2008). *Getting Health Reform Right: A Guide to Improving Performance and Equity*. New York: Oxford University Press.

Rogel, Carol. 1998. *The Breakup of Yugoslavia and the War in Bosnia*. Westport: Greenwood Publishing Group.

Saric, Muhamed, and Victor G. Rodwin. 1993. The Once and Future Health System in the Former Yugoslavia: Myths and Realities. *Journal of Public Health*: 220–237. https://www.nyu.edu/projects/rodwin/future.html.

Savedoff, William D. 2007. What Should a Country Spend on Health Care. *Health Affairs* 26 (4): 962–970. https://www.healthaffairs.org/doi/pdf/10.1377/hlthaff.26.4.962

Segal, Troy. 2019. Diversification. *Investopedia*. Updated Apr 5. https://www.investopedia.com/terms/d/diversification.asp, archived at https://perma.cc/7XED-DSVY

Semiz, Sabina, and Philip C. Aka. 2019. Precision Medicine in the Era of CRISPR-Cas9: Evidence from Bosnia and Herzegovina. *Palgrave Communications*. https://doi.org/10.1057/s41599-019-0346-2.

Share of People Who Smoke Every Day, 1980. to 2012. *Our World in Data*. https://ourworldindata.org/grapher/daily-smoking-prevalence?country=BIH

Slipicević, Osman, and Adisa Malicbegović. 2012. Public and Private Sector[s] in the Health Care System of the Federation [of] Bosnia and Herzegovina: Policy and Strategy. *Materia Socio Medica [Journal of Academy of Medical Sciences of Bosnia and Herzegovina]*, 24(1). doi https://doi.org/10.5455/msm.2012.24.54-57. ncbi.nlm.nih.gov/pmc/articles/PMC3633389/

130    REFERENCES

Slovakia Population 2020. World Population Review. https://worldpopulationre-view.com/countries/slovakia-population/, archived at https://perma.cc/D4GB-77TA

Statute of the Brčko District of Bosnia and Herzegovina. 2000. https://advokat-prnjavorac.com/legislation/Statute-of-the-Brcko-Distrikt-of-Bosnia-and-Herzegovina.pdf

Stern, Alexandra Minna. 2017. *Telling Genes: The Story of Genetic Counseling in America*. Baltimore: Johns Hopkins University Press.

Strong, Carol, et al. 2016. Effects of Adolescent Cigarette Smoking on Adulthood Substance Use and Abuse: The Mediating Role of Educational Attainment. *Substance Use and Misuse* 51 (2): 141–154. https://doi.org/10.310 9/10826084.2015.1073323.

*Summary of the Dayton Peace Agreement on Bosnia and Herzegovina*. 1995. University of Minnesota Human Rights Library. November 30. http://hrli-brary.umn.edu/icty/dayton/daytonsum.html

Tanner, Marcus. 2010. *Croatia: A Nation Forged in War*. 3rd ed. New Haven: Yale University Press.

Toè, Rodolfo. 2016. Census Reveals Bosnia's Changed Demography. *BalkanInsight*, June 30. https://balkaninsight.com/2016/06/30/new-demographic-picture-of-bosnia-finally-revealed-06-30-2016/, archived at https://perma.cc/35DB-T2YZ

UNESCO. *Universal Declaration on Bioethics and Human Rights*. Social and Human Sciences. http://www.unesco.org/new/en/social-and-human-sci-ences/themes/bioethics/bioethics-and-human-rights/, archived at https://perma.cc/F8RH-L82M

UNESCO. Sector for Social and Human Sciences. 2016. *Bioethics Core Curriculum: Section 1: Syllabus Ethics Education Program*. https://unesdoc.unesco.org/ark:/48223/pf0000246885

United Nations Development Program. 2019. *Human Development Report 2019: Beyond Income, Beyond Averages, Beyond Today: Inequalities in Human Development in the 21st Century*. New York: United Nations Development Program.

———. 2020. *COVID-19: Looming Crisis in Developing Countries Threatens to Devastate Economies and Ramp Up Inequality*. March 30. https://www.undp.org/content/undp/en/home/news-centre/news/2020/COVID19_Crisis_in_developing_countries_threatens_devastate_economies.html, archived at https://perma.cc/BJ9P-GYZJ

United Nations High Commissioner for Refugees' Office of the Chief of Mission in Bosnia. 2001. *Health Care in Bosnia and Herzegovina in the Context of the Return of Refugees and Displaced Persons*. Sarajevo. July. https://www.unhcr.org/news/updates/2001/7/3c614f6a4/health-care-bosnia-herzegovina-context-return-refugees-displaced-persons.html

Universal Declaration of Human Rights. 1948. G.A. Res. 217(III)A. (Dec. 10).
Ustav Socijalisticke Federativne Republike Jugoslvije [Constitution of the Socialist Federal Republic of Yugoslavia]. 1974. Translated in *Constitution of the Socialist Federal Republic of Yugoslavia*. World Statesmen.org. http://www.worldstatesmen.org/Yugoslavia-Constitution1974.pdf. Last visited 25 Mar 2020.
Varga, Orsolya, and Jorge Sequeiros. Definitions of Genetic Testing in European and Other Legal Documents. *EuroGentist*. http://www.eurogentest.org/index.php?id=732, archived at https://perma.cc/S6RT-YYUU
Venice Commission. 2012. *Opinion on Legal Certainty and the Independence of the Judiciary in Bosnia and Herzegovina*. Opinion No. 648/2011 June 8.
Vienna Convention on the Law of Treaties. 1969. 1115 U.N.T.S. 331. May 23. https://treaties.un.org/doc/Publication/UNTS/Volume%201155/volume-1155-I-18232-English.pdf
Wallace, Rebecca M.M., and Olga Martin-Ortega. 2013. *International Law*. 7th ed. London: Sweet & Maxwell.
West Virginia Population (Demographics, Maps, Graphs) 2020. World Population Review. https://worldpopulationreview.com/states/west-virginia-population/, archived at https://perma.cc/SM7M-28PW
What Are Genome Editing and CRISPR-Cas9?. *U.S. National Library of Medicine: Genetics Home Reference*. https://ghr.nlm.nih.gov/primer/genomicresearch/genomeediting, archived at https://perma.cc/F4T8-L2VK
What Is Bioethics. *Center for Practical Ethics*. https://practicalbioethics.org/what-is-bioethics
What Is DNA?. *US National Library of Medicine: Genetics Home Reference*. https://ghr.nlm.nih.gov/primer/basics/dna, archived at https://perma.cc/AA63-M7JP
What Is EuroGentest. *European Society of Human Genetics (ESHG)*. http://www.eurogentest.org/index.php?id=160, archived at https://perma.cc/B9PM-KPWW
What Is Genome Editing?. *YourGenome*. https://www.yourgenome.org/facts/what-is-genome-editing, archived at https://perma.cc/7JZ3-TUZV
Wilson, Frank L. 1996. *Concepts and Issues in Comparative Politics: An Introduction*. Upper Saddle River: Prentice Hall.
Wolff, Jonathan. 2017 (2013). Karl Marx. *Stanford Encyclopedia of Philosophy*. 26 August 2013. Revised 12 April 2017. https://plato.stanford.edu/entries/marx/
World Bank. 2012. *Smoking: An Endemic Problem in Bosnia and Herzegovina*. November 20. http://www.worldbank.org/en/news/feature/2012/11/20/smoking-an-endemic-problem-in-bosnia-and-herzegovina, archived at https://perma.cc/H4YJ-H9U6
———. 2017. *Life Expectancy at Birth, Total (Years)*. https://data.worldbank.org/indicator/SP.DYN.LE00.IN, archived at https://perma.cc/9J9R-4SX8

———. *Health Expenditure Total (% of GDP)*. https://data.worldbank.org/indicator/SH.XPD.TOTL.ZS

World Federation of Hemophilia. 2011. *Report on the Annual Global Survey*. December. https://www1.wfh.org/publication/files/pdf-1427.pdf

World Health Organization. 1978. *Declaration of Alma Ata, International Conference on PHC [Primary Health Care]*. Alma-Ata: USSR. 6–12 September. http://www.who.int/publications/almaata_declaration_en.pdf

———. 1995. *World Health Report 1995: Bridging the Gaps*. Geneva: World Health Organization. https://www.who.int/whr/1995/en/whr95_en.pdf?ua=1

———. 2000. *The World Health Report 2000: Health Systems: Improving Performance*. Geneva: World Health Organization.

———. 2010. *The World Health Report: Health Systems Financing: The Path to Universal Coverage*. Geneva: World Health Organization.

———. 2011a. *The Abuja Declaration: Ten Years On*. https://www.who.int/healthsystems/publications/abuja_declaration/en/

———. 2011b. *World Report on Disability*. Geneva: World Health Organization. who.int/disabilities/world_report/2011/report.pdf.

———. 2014. *Health in All Policies: Helsinki Statement Framework for Country Action*. Geneva: World Health Organization.

———. 2015. *The Global Prevalence of Anaemia in 2011*. Geneva: World Health Organization.

———. 2020. *Q&A on Coronaviruses (COVID-19)*. April 17. who.int/newsroom/q-a-detail/q-a-coronaviruses, archived at https://perma.cc/3UNS-L92T

———. *About WHO*. http://www.who.int/about/en/, archived at https://perma.cc/9RSG-VFQ4

———. *Bosnia and Herzegovina*. who.int/countries/bih/en/, archived at https://perma.cc/WF8R-233D

———. *What Is Universal Coverage?* http://www.who.int/health_financing/universal_coverage_definition/en/

———. *The Molecular Genetic Epidemiology of Cystic Fibrosis*. https://www.who.int/genomics/publications/en/HGN_WB_04.02_fig 2.pdf

———. *What Is Health Financing for Universal Coverage?* http://www.who.int/health_financing/universal_coverage_definition/en/, archived at https://perma.cc/5ADD-24QK

———. *Metrics: Disability-Adjusted Life Years (DALY)*. https://www.who.int/healthinfo/global_burden_disease/metrics_daly/en/

The World Health Organization's Ranking of the World's Health Systems, by Rank. *Countries of the World*. photius.com/rankings/healthranks.html

World Health Organization. Regional Office for Europe. 2016. *Tobacco Control Fact Sheet: Bosnia and Herzegovina*.

Yakob, Bereket, and Busisiwe Purity Ncama. 2017. Measuring Health System Responsiveness at Facility Level in Ethiopia: Performance, Correlates[,] and Implications. *BMC Health Service Research* 17: 263. https://doi.org/10.1186/s12913-017-2224-1.

Yee, Hoi Mun. 2017. Bosnia's Roma Try to Break Out of Isolation. *Balkan Insight*. June 14. https://balkaninsight.com/2017/06/14/bosnia-s-roma-try-to-break-out-of-isolation-06-13-2017-2/

Zimmerman, Mary Ko. 2020. Comparative Health-Care Systems. *Encyclopedia of Sociology*. (Updated Jan 25). https://www.encyclopedia.com/social-sciences/encyclopedias-almanacs-transcripts-and-maps/comparative-health-care-systems

Živković, Andreja. 2017. Analysis on Tax Justice: Bosnia and Herzegovina. *Balkan Monitoring Public Finances*. September. http://wings-of-hope.ba/wp-content/uploads/2016/12/D3.4.3.1.-Analysis-on-Tax-Justice-Bosnia-and-Herzegovina.pdf

Zuniga, José M., et al., eds. 2013. *Advancing the Human Right to Health*. New York: Oxford University Press.

# Index[1]

[1] Note: Page numbers followed by 'n' refer to notes.

© The Author(s) 2020
P. C. Aka, *Genetic Counseling and Preventive Medicine in Post-War Bosnia*, https://doi.org/10.1007/978-981-15-7987-5